Nutrition Support

Nutrition Power to Eat, to Learn

Emy Reed

2020

TABLE OF CONTENTS

CHAPTER ONE

INTRODUCTION

Nutrition is the science that interprets the connection of supplements and different substances in nourishment in connection to upkeep, development, multiplication, health and illness of a creature. It incorporates nourishment consumption, retention, absorption, biosynthesis, catabolism and excretion. The eating routine of a life form is the thing that it eats, which is to a great extent dictated by the accessibility and attractiveness of nourishments. For people, a solid eating regimen incorporates arrangement of nourishment and capacity techniques that safeguard supplements from oxidation, warmth or filtering, and that lessens danger of foodborne ailments. In people, an undesirable eating regimen can cause lack related infections, for example, visual impairment, iron deficiency, scurvy, preterm birth, stillbirth and cretinism, or supplement overabundance health undermining conditions, for example, obesity and metabolic syndrome; and such basic incessant foundational illnesses as cardiovascular disease, diabetes, and osteoporosis. Undernutrition can prompt squandering in intense cases, and the hindering of marasmus in interminable instances of malnutrition. The main recorded dietary exhortation, cut into a Babylonian stone tablet in around 2500 BC, forewarned those with torment inside to abstain from eating onions for three days. Scurvy, later saw as a Vitamin C lack, was first portrayed in 1500 BC in the Ebers Papyrus. As indicated by Walter Gratzer, the investigation of nourishment most likely started during the sixth century BC. In China, the idea of qi built up, a soul or "wind" like what Western Europeans later called pneuma. Food was ordered into "hot" (for instance, meats, blood, ginger, and hot flavors) and "cold" (green vegetables) in China, India, Malaya, and Persia. Humors grew maybe first in China close by qi. Ho the Physician presumed that ailments are brought about by insufficiencies of components (Wu Xing: fire, water, earth, wood, and metal), and he arranged ailments just as endorsed diets. About a similar time in Italy, Alcmaeon of Croton (a Greek) composed of the significance of harmony between what goes in and what goes out, and cautioned that irregularity would bring about ailment set apart by heftiness or cmaciation. The primary recorded healthful test with human subjects is found in the Bible's Book of Daniel. Daniel and his companions were caught by the lord of

Babylon during an intrusion of Israel. Chosen as court workers, they were to partake in the ruler's fine nourishments and wine. Be that as it may, they protested, favoring vegetables (heartbeats) and water as per their Jewish dietary limitations. The ruler's central steward hesitantly consented to a preliminary. Daniel and his companions got their eating routine for ten days and were then contrasted with the lord's men. Seeming more advantageous, they were permitted to proceed with their diet.Around 475 BC, Anaxagoras expressed that nourishment is consumed by the human body and, in this manner, contains "homeomerics" (generative parts), proposing the presence of nutrients. Around 400 BC, Hippocrates, who perceived and was worried about heftiness, which may have been regular in southern Europe at the time, stated, "Let nourishment be your prescription and drug be your food." The works that are still ascribed to him, Corpus Hippocraticum, called for control and stressed exercise. During the 1500s, Paracelsus was most likely the first to reprimand Galen publicly. Also in the sixteenth century, researcher and craftsman Leonardo da Vinci contrasted digestion with a consuming flame. Leonardo didn't distribute his takes a shot at this subject, yet he was not terrified of having an independent perspective and he certainly couldn't help contradicting Galen. Ultimately, sixteenth century works of Andreas Vesalius, here and there called the dad of present day human life structures, upset Galen's ideas. He was trailed by puncturing thought amalgamated with the time's otherworldliness and religion now and again powered by the mechanics of Newton and Galileo. Jan Baptist van Helmont, who found a few gases, for example, carbon dioxide, played out the primary quantitative test. Robert Boyle propelled science. Sanctorius estimated body weight. Doctor Herman Boerhaave demonstrated the stomach related procedure. Physiologist Albrecht von Haller worked out the distinction among nerves and muscles.At times overlooked during his life, James Lind, a doctor in the British naval force, played out the main logical sustenance test in 1747. Lind found that lime juice spared mariners that had been adrift for a considerable length of time from scurvy, a destructive and difficult draining issue. Somewhere in the range of 1500 and 1800, an expected 2,000,000 mariners had passed on of scurvy. The revelation was disregarded for a long time, after which British mariners got known as "limeys." The basic Vitamin C inside citrus natural products would not be distinguished by researchers until 1932.

CHAPTER TWO

WHAT ARE NUTRIENTS?

The list of supplements that individuals are known to require is, in the expressions of Marion Nestle, "very likely incomplete". As of 2014, supplements are believed to be of two sorts: macronutrients which are required in moderately huge sums, and micronutrients which are required in littler quantities. A kind of sugar, dietary fiber, for example non-edible material, for example, cellulose, is required, for both mechanical and biochemical reasons, in spite of the fact that the precise reasons stay vague. A few supplements can be put away - the fat-solvent vitamins - while others are required pretty much constantly. Unexpected weakness can be brought about by an absence of required supplements, or for certain vitamins and minerals, an over the top required supplement.

Nourishment is the study of nourishment and its relationship to wellbeing – how the human body utilizes nourishment and procedures the supplements it contains to empower the body to perform capacities (for example the heart to thump, the lungs to inhale, the kidneys to channel blood, the mind to think and so forth.). Incorporated in this definition is how a lot of vitality (kilojoules) a body needs to keep up a solid weight. Vitality is conveyed to the body through nourishments. Any vitality expended (as starches, protein or fat) and not utilized for digestion, development or physical movement will be put away as muscle versus fat. There are numerous components that direct how much vitality an individual needs, however in straightforward terms the more the body moves, the more noteworthy the measure of vitality will be required. A supplement is a source of sustenance, a part of nourishment, for example, protein, sugar, fat, Vitamin, mineral, fiber, and water.

- Macronutrients are supplements we need in generally enormous amounts.

- Micronutrients are supplements we need in generally little amounts.

Macronutrients can be additionally part into vitality macronutrients (that give vitality), and macroVitamins that don't give vitality. Vitality macronutrients give vitality, which is estimated either in kilocalories (kcal or calories) or Joules. 1 kilocalorie (calorie) = 4185.8 joules. The compelling administration of nourishment admission and sustenance are both key to great health. Brilliant sustenance and nourishment decisions can help avert infection. Eating the correct nourishments can enable your body to adapt all the more effectively to a continuous sickness. Seeing great sustenance and focusing on what you eat can assist you with keeping up or improve your health. Nourishment and sustenance are the manner in which that we get fuel, giving vitality to our bodies. We have to supplant supplements in our bodies with another inventory each day. Water is a significant segment of nourishment. Fats, proteins, and sugars are altogether required. Keeping up key Vitamins and minerals are likewise essential to keeping up great health. For pregnant ladies and grown-ups more than 50, Vitamins, for example, Vitamin D and minerals, for example, calcium and iron are essential to think about when picking nourishments to eat, just as conceivable dietary enhancements. A sound eating routine incorporates a great deal of regular nourishments. A sizeable bit of a solid eating regimen should comprise of foods grown from the ground, particularly ones that are red, orange, or dim green. Entire grains, for example, entire wheat and dark colored rice, ought to likewise have an impact in your eating regimen. For grown-ups, dairy items ought to be non-fat or low-fat. Protein can comprise of lean meat and poultry, fish, eggs, beans, vegetables, and soy items, for example, tofu, just as unsalted seeds and nuts. Great sustenance additionally includes evading particular sorts of nourishments. Sodium is utilized intensely in prepared nourishments and is risky for individuals with hypertension. The USDA encourages grown-ups to devour under 300 milligrams (mg) every day of cholesterol (found in meat and full-fat dairy items among others). Singed nourishment, strong fats, and trans fats found in margarine and prepared nourishments can be hurtful to heart health. Refined grains (a health doctor flour, a health doctor rice) and refined sugar (table sugar, high fructose corn syrup) are likewise terrible for long haul health, particularly in individuals with diabetes. Liquor can be perilous to health in sums more than one serving for every day for a lady and two every day for a man. There are some top notch, free rules accessible for good dieting plans that give more subtleties on parcel size, complete calorie utilization, what to eat a greater amount of, and what to eat less of to get solid and remain as such. Nutrients, sustenance, or nourishment, is the stock of materials - nourishment - required by creatures and cells to remain alive. In science and human prescription, sustenance is the science or practice of expending and using nourishments. In medical clinics, nourishment may allude to the nourishment prerequisites of patients, including healthful arrangements conveyed through an IV (intravenous) or IG (intragastric) tube. Healthful science contemplates how the body separates nourishment (catabolism) and how it fixes and makes cells and tissue (anabolism). Catabolism and anabolism joined can likewise be alluded to as digestion. Nourishing science additionally analyzes how the body reacts to nourishment. The human body requires seven significant sorts of supplements. Not all supplements give vitality but rather are as yet significant, for example, water and fiber. Micronutrients are significant however required in littler sums. Vitamins are basic natural aggravates that the human body can't combine. As atomic science, organic chemistry, and hereditary qualities advance, nourishment has gotten increasingly centered around digestion and metabolic pathways - biochemical strides through which substances inside us are changed starting with one structure then onto the next. Nourishment additionally centers around how ailments, conditions, and issues can be anticipated or decreased with a sound eating routine.

Additionally, sustenance includes recognizing how certain illnesses and conditions might be brought about by dietary components, for example, terrible eating routine (lack of healthy sustenance), nourishment hypersensitivities, and nourishment bigotries.

Dietitian versus nutritionist

An enrolled dietitian nutritionist (RD or RDN) examines nourishment, sustenance, and dietetics through an authorize college and endorsed educational plan, at that point finishes a thorough temporary position and breezes through a licensure test to turn into an enlisted dietitian. A nutritionist (without the title of a RD or RDN) considers sustenance by means of self-study or through proper training however doesn't meet the necessities to utilize the titles RD or RDN. The two terms are frequently compatible, yet they are not indistinguishable.

Dietetics

Dietetics is the translation and correspondence of the study of sustenance; it assists individuals with settling on educated and commonsense decisions about nourishment and way of life in both health and sickness. Some portion of a dietician's course incorporates both medical clinic and network settings. Dietitians work in an assortment of zones, from private practice to human services, instruction, corporate health, and research, while an a lot littler extent work in the nourishment business. A dietitian must have a perceived qualification or postgraduate certificate in nourishment and dietetics and meet proceeding with training necessities to fill in as a dietitian. Nutritionists at times complete research for nourishment producers. Sustenance is the investigation of supplements in nourishment, how the body utilizes supplements, and the connection between diet, health, and disease. Significant nourishment makers utilize nutritionists and nourishment researchers. Nutritionists may likewise work in news-casting, training, and research. Numerous nutritionists work in the field of nourishment science and innovation. There is a ton of cover between what nutritionists and dietitians do and study. A few nutritionists work in a medicinal services setting, a few dietitians work in the nourishment business, yet a higher level of nutritionists work in the nourishment business and in nourishment science and innovation, and a higher level of dietitians work in human services, corporate health, research, and instruction. There are six fundamental supplements that the body needs to work appropriately. Supplements are mixes in nourishments fundamental to life and wellbeing, furnishing us with vitality, the structure hinders for fix and development and substances important to direct concoction forms.

There are six significant supplements: Carbohydrates (CHO), Lipids (fats), Proteins, Vitamins, Minerals, Water. Taking a gander at the AGHE, what nutrition classes are the essential wellsprings of every one of the accompanying ?

- Proteins: meat, dairy, vegetables, nuts, fish and eggs

- Starches: pasta, rice, oats, breads, potatoes, milk, natural product, sugar

- Lipids (most ordinarily called fats): oils, spread, margarine, nuts, seeds, avocados and olives, meat and fish

- Nutrients: regular nutrients incorporate the water dissolvable B vitamins and vitamin C and the fat solvent vitamins A, D, E and K

- Water as a source of cell hydration.

Foods grown from the ground are commonly great sources of Vitamin C and An and folic corrosive (a B bunch nutrient). Grains and oats are commonly great wellsprings of the B bunch nutrients and fiber. Full-fat dairy and egg yolks are for the most part wellsprings of the fat dissolvable nutrients A, D and E. Milk and vegetable or soya bean oil are commonly great wellsprings of nutrient K, which can likewise be orchestrated by gut microscopic organisms.

Minerals: (sodium, calcium, iron, iodine, magnesium, and so on.): all nourishments contain some type of minerals. Milk and dairy items are a decent wellspring of calcium and magnesium. Red meat is a decent wellspring of iron and zinc. Fish and vegetables (contingent upon the dirt in which they are delivered) are commonly great wellsprings of iodine

Water: As a refreshment and a segment of numerous nourishments, particularly vegetables and natural products.

The kilojoule is the proportion of vitality utilized in Australia. It is the International unit for vitality, however a few nations (for example USA) still utilize the calorie. The transformation is: 4.2kJ = 1 calorie. We use it to decide how a lot of vitality a nourishment will give when we eat it.

The supplements that give vitality are normally alluded to as macronutrients (sugars, lipids, and proteins). Starches and proteins give a comparative measure of vitality per gram of nourishment. Lipids are a concentrated wellspring of vitality and give double the measure of vitality than that provided by proteins and starches.

For your data as it were:

- CHOs = 16 kJ per gram of CHO

- Protein = 17 kJ per gram of protein

- Lipids = 37 kJ per gram of lipid

Kids matured between 4-18 years require ~6500 to 14000 kJ every day. The estimated number of kilojoules a youngster devours every day will rely upon their age and physical action level. The qualities given are for normal physical action as it were. For additional data, it would be ideal if you allude to the Nutrient Reference Values for Australia.

CHAPTER THREE

MACRONUTRIENTS

The macronutrients are starches, fiber, fats, protein, and water. The macronutrients (barring fiber and water) give auxiliary material (amino acids from which proteins are manufactured, and lipids from which cell films and some flagging particles are assembled) and vitality. A portion of the basic material can be utilized to create vitality inside, and in either case it is estimated in Joules or kilocalories (regularly called "Calories" and composed with a capital C to separate them from little 'c' calories). Sugars and proteins give 17 kJ around (4 kcal) of vitality per gram, while fats give 37 kJ (9 kcal) per gram, however the net vitality from either relies upon such factors as retention and stomach related exertion, which shift significantly from example to occurrence. Vitamins, minerals, fiber, and water don't give vitality, however are required for different reasons.

Particles of sugars and fats comprise of carbon, hydrogen, and oxygen iotas. Sugars extend from straightforward monosaccharides (glucose, fructose and galactose) to complex polysaccharides (starch). Fats are triglycerides, made of arranged unsaturated fat monomers bound to a glycerol spine. Some unsaturated fats, however not all, are fundamental in the eating regimen: they can't be combined in the body. Protein particles contain nitrogen iotas notwithstanding carbon, oxygen, and hydrogen. The major segments of protein are nitrogen-containing amino acids, some of which are basic as in people can't make them inside. A portion of the amino acids are convertible (with the use of vitality) to glucose and can be utilized for vitality generation, similarly as normal glucose, in a procedure known as gluconeogenesis. By separating existing protein, the carbon skeleton of the different amino acids can be processed to intermediates in cell breath; the rest of the smelling salts is disposed of fundamentally as urea in urine.

What are macronutrients?

The human body and the entirety of its amazing components are very mind boggling, implying that it requires an assortment of supplements so as to work ideally. What we eat is fundamental for addressing these requirements. Macronutrients help us develop, create, fix, give us vitality, and make us feel better. They each have their own job and capacities in the body. Macronutrients allude to the three fundamental segments of each diet — sugars, fat, and protein — with a reward fourth, water. Full scale, signifying "enormous," insinuates the way that these supplements are required in bigger amounts. Pretty much every nourishment has a mix of macroVitamins, however the distinction lies in the piece of these macronutrients. The macronutrients that has the most noteworthy rate in every nourishment will decide how it is arranged, for example as protein, carb or fat. For example, avocados comprise of about 70% fat, 8% carb, and 2% protein, so despite the fact that they contain a portion of different macros, they would be named a fat. Another model would be an apple which comprises of about 95% carb, 2% protein, and 3% fat. In the event that you didn't get it as of now, that suppers apples are named a carbohydrate.

Rundown on types macronutrients:

Carbohydrates

Carbohydrates are comprised of chains of starch and sugar that the body separates into glucose. These are the body's fundamental source of vitality and the cerebrum's essential source. This is imperative to know in light of the fact that, since your mind requires fuel consistently so as to work, your body is extremely proficient at putting away glucose (as glycogen) in the liver and muscles. Sugars of about 4 kcal per gram is required. Sugar particles incorporate monosaccharides (glucose, fructose, galactose), disaccharides, and polysaccharides (starch). Healthfully, polysaccharides are supported over monosaccharides since they are increasingly mind boggling and along these lines take more time to separate and be ingested into the circulation system; this implies they don't cause significant spikes in glucose levels, which are connected to heart and vascular infections.

Great sources of sugars:

- Entire grains (darker and wild rice, oats, amaranth, entire wheat)

- Bland vegetables (potatoes, sweet potatoes, corn, beets)

- Vegetables (beans, lentils, chickpeas, peas)

- Natural products (apple, oranges, berries, pear, banana)

Fats

Fats are required for mental health, making

hormones and supporting in the assimilation of fat-dissolvable Vitamins (A, D, E, K). They have the most significant carbohydrate level per gram, implying that they require more vitality to consume, and yet, are useful for expanding sentiments of satiety, which means they will keep you more full for more.

Great sources of fat:

- Avocado and avocado oil

- Olives and olive oil

- Full-fat dairy and natural, grass-nourished spread

- Nuts (almonds, pecans, cashews)

- Seeds (chia, pumpkin, flax)

- fatty fish (salmon or trout)

Protein

Protein gives amino acids, which are the structure squares of cell and muscle structure. Altogether, there are 20 sorts of amino acids, nine of which are basic, implying that your body requires them from nourishment. Protein in the body is utilized past simply muscle — it is the center part of organs, bones, hair, compounds, and all tissue. Protein likewise helps bolster a solid invulnerable framework. Proteins of about 4 kcal per gram is required for human sustenance.There are 20 amino acids - natural mixes found in nature that consolidate to shape proteins. Some amino acids are fundamental, which means they should be expended. Other amino acids are unimportant on the grounds that the body can make them.

Great sources of protein (natural liked):

- Fish and fish (salmon, fish, a health doctor fish, shrimp, crab, shellfish)

- Poultry (chicken and turkey)

- Lean and natural meat (pork, hamburger, sheep)

- Eggs

- Dairy (insignificantly prepared cheddar, unsweetened yogurt, and non-dairy options)

- Tofu and soy items (negligibly prepared)

Water

Water doesn't contain any calories or supplements,

however it is as yet viewed as a macroVitamin since we require it in huge sums. Indeed, water makes up a huge bit of our bodies. It fills in as a transporter, carrying supplements to cells and expelling squanders. It controls our internal heat level and aids digestion. The Institute of Medicine prescribes around 13 cups of water (around three liters) for men and around nine cups (or 2.2 liters) for ladies. Be that as it may, this can fluctuate as indicated by movement level, condition, ailments, and liquor utilization (which is drying out). Not certain in the event that you get enough water? Perhaps the most ideal ways is to trace it.Liquor is likewise viewed as a macronutrient since it contains a weighty 7 calories for every gram. It isn't fundamental to have in your eating routine, yet in the event that you discover satisfaction in having a glass every once in a while, practice balance and go for solid choices.

Macronutrients proportions

Since we've replied, What are macronutrients?, we should discuss perfect large scale proportion ranges. Much the same as diet and wellness, macronutrients proportions are not one-size-fits-all. There is no perfect macronutrients proportion that suits everybody and your needs will change as indicated by various factors throughout your life. A few people may improve on a lower starch diet, while another person may feel more invigorated on a higher fat eating routine. As a rule, mean to have more carbohydrates when that you're progressively dynamic and in case you're stationary, you may see better outcomes on a higher protein feast plan. Another explanation we don't suggest a quite certain macronutrients proportion is that it doesn't utter a word about the nature of the supplements. A proportion just considers the quantity of macroVitamins which implies that carbohydrates from a health doctor sugar and quinoa are taken care of a similar way. The best thing you can do is...

- Concentrate on balance

- Organize entire nourishments

- Watch your segment sizes

Attempting distinctive macroVitamin targets enables you to figure out which levels work best for you. These reaches can differ contingent upon which kind of diet you are traceing. Here are a few instances of full scale ranges:

Standard eating routine macros extend:

- Protein: 10-35% of calories

- carbohydrates: 45-65% of calories

- Fat: 20-35% of calories

Low-carbohydrate diet macros extend:

- Protein: 20-30% of calories

- carbohydrates: 30-40% of calories

- Fat: 30-40% of calories

Keto diet macros go:

- Protein: 20-25% of calories

- carbohydrates: 5-10% of calories

- Fat: 70-75% of calories

Macronutrients adding calculator: How to ascertain macronutrients

Time to put our geek tops on! A calorie is a unit used to quantify the vitality delivering estimation of nourishment however this isn't the most precise measure. To get specialized, a calorie is characterized as the measure of warmth important to raise the temperature of one gram of water, one degree centigrade.

Each macronutrients has an alternate calorie level for each gram weight.

- Starch = 4 calories for each gram

- Protein = 4 calories for each gram

- Fat = 9 calories for each gram

The all out calorie substance of nourishment relies upon the measure of starch, protein, and fat it contains. As should be obvious, fat is the most thought source of vitality, yielding 9 kcal per gram. This is the place those old school low-fats eats less carbohydrates began. The thinking depended on the thought that on the off chance that you expel the more unhealthy per gram macroVitamin, it is simpler to decrease the volume of nourishment. In any case, this is defective since fat is in reality very satisfying and can help advance weight reduction when eaten with some restraint.

Nourishment certainties mark

Nourishment data is regularly recorded in grams,

however we'll show you a little stunt that will make you a Macro Master. Essentially increase the grams of every full scale by the quantity of calories per gram. At that point, add these numbers together to decide the all out calories in a thing.

Here's a model, say you realize that a granola bar has:

- Absolute fat: 6g

- Complete starch: 25g

- Protein: 10g

Presently we should connect it to the calorie level per gram, of each macronutrients... .

- Fat: 6g x 9kcal per gram = 54kcal

- Sugar: 25g x 4kcal per gram = 100kcal

- Protein: 10g x 4kcal per gram = 40kcal

Recollect that calories are normally adjusted so the qualities may not generally be precise. This makes the complete calories around 194 kcal. Prepare to be blown away. This health bar isn't even solid by any means! Its principle source of starch is from sugar! This is the reason it's constantly critical to check the nourishment name.

CHAPTER FOUR

CARBOHYDRATES

Starches might be named monosaccharides, disaccharides, or polysaccharides relying upon the quantity of monomer (sugar) units they contain. They establish an enormous piece of nourishments, for example, rice, noodles, bread, and other grain-based items, likewise potatoes, yams, beans, organic products, natural product juices and vegetables. Monosaccharides, disaccharides, and polysaccharides contain one, two, and at least three sugar units, separately. Polysaccharides are frequently alluded to as unpredictable starches since they are ordinarily long, various stretched chains of sugar units. Generally, basic sugars are accepted to be retained rapidly, and in this way to raise blood-glucose levels more quickly than complex starches. This, notwithstanding, isn't accurate. Some straightforward starches (e.g., fructose) pursue distinctive metabolic pathways (e.g., fructolysis) that outcome in just a fractional catabolism to glucose, while, fundamentally, numerous mind boggling sugars might be processed at a similar rate as basic carbohydrates. The World Health Organization (WHO) suggests that additional sugars ought to speak to close to 10% of all out vitality intake.Starch devoured in nourishment yields 3.87 kilocalories of vitality per gram for straightforward sugars, and 3.57 to 4.12 kilocalories per gram for complex carb in most other foods. Relatively significant levels of sugar are related with prepared food sources or refined nourishments produced using plants, including desserts, treats and sweet, table sugar, nectar, sodas, breads and wafers, sticks and natural product items, pastas and breakfast oats. Lower measures of starch are normally connected with foul nourishments, including beans, tubers, rice, and grungy fruit. Animal-based food sources by and large have the most reduced sugar levels, in spite of the fact that milk contains a high extent of lactose. Living beings ordinarily can't process a wide range of sugar to yield vitality. Glucose is an about all inclusive and available source of vitality. Numerous living beings likewise can process different monosaccharides and disaccharides yet glucose is frequently used first. In Escherichia coli, for instance, the lac operon will express proteins for the absorption of lactose when it is available, however in the event that both lactose and glucose are available the lac operon is quelled, bringing about the glucose being utilized first (see: Diauxie). Polysaccharides are likewise regular sources of vitality. Numerous life forms can undoubtedly separate starches into glucose; most life forms, in any case, can't process cellulose or different polysaccharides like chitin and arabinoxylans. These starch types can be processed by certain microorganisms and protists. Ruminants and termites, for instance, use microorganisms to process cellulose. Despite the fact that these mind boggling starches are not entirely edible, they speak to a significant dietary component for people, called dietary fiber. Fiber improves processing, among other benefits. The Institute of Medicine suggests that American and Canadian grown-ups get between 45–65% of dietary vitality from entire grain carbohydrates. The Food and Agriculture Organization and World Health Organization mutually prescribe that national dietary rules set an objective of 55–75% of all out vitality from starches, however just 10% legitimately from sugars (their term for straightforward carbohydrates). A 2017 Cochrane Systematic Review reasoned that there was inadequate proof to help the case that entire grain diets can influence cardiovascular disease. Nutritionists frequently allude to starches as either basic or complex. Be that as it may, the accurate differentiation between these gatherings can be uncertain. The term complex sugar was first utilized in the U.S. Senate Select Committee on Nutrition and Human Needs production Dietary Goals for the United States (1977) where it was proposed to recognize sugars from different starches (which were seen to be healthfully superior). However, the report put "natural product, vegetables and entire grains" in the perplexing carb section, regardless of the way that these may contain sugars just as polysaccharides. This disarray continues as today a few nutritionists utilize the term complex starch to allude to any kind of absorbable saccharide present in an entire nourishment, where fiber, Vitamins and minerals are likewise found (instead of handled sugars, which give vitality however hardly any different supplements). The standard use, in any case, is to arrange starches synthetically: straightforward on the off chance that they are sugars (monosaccharides and disaccharides) and complex in the event that they are polysaccharides (or oligosaccharides). Regardless, the basic versus complex compound differentiation has little an incentive for deciding the nourishing nature of carbohydrates. Some straightforward starches (for example fructose) raise blood glucose gradually, while some perplexing carbohydrates (starches), particularly whenever prepared, raise glucose quickly.

The surined of assimilation is dictated by an assortment of elements including which different supplements are overcome with the starch, how the nourishment is readied, singular contrasts in digestion, and the science of the carbohydrate. The USDA's Dietary Guidelines for Americans 2010 call for moderate-to high-starch utilization from a fair diet that incorporates six one-ounce servings of grain nourishments every day, in any event half from entire grain sources and the rest from enriched. The glycemic list (GI) and glycemic load ideas have been created to portray nourishment conduct during human assimilation. They rank starch rich nourishments dependent on the rate and extent of their impact on blood glucose levels. Glycemic list is a proportion of how rapidly nourishment glucose is consumed, while glycemic load is a proportion of the all out absorbable glucose in food sources. The insulin record is a comparable, later order technique that positions nourishments dependent on their consequences for blood insulin levels, which are brought about by glucose (or starch) and some amino acids in nourishment.

HEALTH IMPACTS OF DIETARY SUGAR

Low-sugar diet

Low-sugar diets may miss the health points of interest –, for example, expanded admission of dietary fiber – managed by great starches found in vegetables and heartbeats, entire grains, natural products, and vegetables. Disadvantages of the eating regimen may incorporate halitosis, migraine and blockage, and when all is said in done the potential unfriendly impacts of sugar confined weight control plans are under-looked into, especially for potential dangers of osteoporosis and malignant growth incidence. Starch limited eating regimens can be as successful as low-fat eating regimens in accomplishing weight reduction over the transient when in general calorie admission is reduced. An Endocrine Society logical explanation said that "when calorie admission is held consistent [...] muscle to fat ratio aggregation doesn't give off an impression of being influenced by even extremely articulated changes in the measure of fat versus sugar in the diet." In the long haul, viable weight reduction or upkeep relies upon calorie restriction, not the proportion of macroVitamins in a diet. The thinking of diet advocates that carbohydrates cause undue fat amassing by expanding blood insulin levels, and that low-carb slims down have a "metabolic bit of leeway", isn't bolstered by clinical evidence. Further, it isn't clear how low-carb eating less junk food influences cardiovascular health, albeit two surveys demonstrated that carb limitation may improve lipid markers of cardiovascular sickness risk. Starch confined eating regimens are not any more compelling than a regular sound eating routine in avoiding the beginning of type 2 diabetes, yet for individuals with type 2 diabetes, they are a feasible choice for getting more fit or assisting with glycemic control. There is restricted proof to help routine utilization of low-sugar eating less junk food in overseeing type 1 diabetes. The American Diabetes Association prescribes that individuals with diabetes ought to embrace a for the most part solid eating regimen, instead of an eating regimen concentrated on carb or other macronutrients. An outrageous type of low-starch diet – the ketogenic diet – is built up as a restorative eating routine for treating epilepsy. Through big name support during the mid 21st century, it turned into a prevailing fashion diet as a methods for weight reduction, yet with dangers of bothersome symptoms, for example, low vitality levels and expanded yearning, a sleeping disorder, queasiness, and gastrointestinal discomfort.[43] The British Dietetic Association named it one of the "best 5 most exceedingly terrible celeb diets to maintain a strategic distance from in 2018". Starches are the sugars, starches and filaments found in natural products, grains, vegetables and milk items. In spite of the fact that regularly defamed in vogue slims down, sugars — one of the essential nutrition classes — are critical to a solid eating routine. "Starches are macronutrients, which means they are one of the three primary ways the body acquires vitality, or calories," said Paige Smathers, an Utah-based enrolled dietitian. The American Diabetes Association noticed that sugars are the body's primary source of vitality. They are called sugars on the grounds that, at the concoction level, they contain carbon, hydrogen and oxygen. There are three macronutrients: starches, protein and fats, Smathers said. Macronutrients are fundamental for legitimate body working, and the body requires a lot of them. All macroVitamins must be gotten through diet; the body can't create macroVitamins all alone. The prescribed day by day sum (RDA) of carbohydrates for grown-ups is 135 grams, as per the National Institutes of Health (NIH); in any case, the NIH likewise suggests that everybody ought to have their very own sugar objective. Carb consumption for the vast majority ought to be somewhere in the range of 45% and 65% of all out calories. One gram of sugars approaches around 4 calories, so an eating routine of 1,800 calories for every day would rise to around 202 grams on the low end and 292 grams of carbohydrates on the very good quality. Notwithstanding, individuals with diabetes ought not eat in excess of 200 grams of carbohydrates every day, while pregnant ladies need at any rate 175 grams.

Capacity of starches

Starches give fuel to the focal sensory system and vitality for working muscles. They likewise keep protein from being utilized as a vitality source and empower fat digestion, according to Iowa State University. Likewise, "sugars are significant for cerebrum work," Smathers said. They are an effect on "temperament, memory, and so forth., just as a surinedy vitality source." truth be told, the RDA of starches depends on the measure of carbohydrates the mind needs to work. Two ongoing investigations distributed in the diary Proceedings of the National Academy of Sciences have likewise connected carbohydrates to basic leadership. In the examinations, individuals who had a high-starch breakfast were less ready to share when playing the "final proposal game" than the individuals who ate high-protein morning meals. Researchers conjecture this might be brought about by benchmark dopamine levels, which are higher subsequent to eating starches. This doesn't mean carbohydrates make you mean, however underscores how various sorts of nourishment admission can influence discernment and conduct.

Simple sugars versus Complex sugars

Sugars are delegated straightforward or complex, Smathers said. The contrast between the two structures is the synthetic structure and how rapidly the sugar is consumed and processed. As a rule, basic carbohydrates are processed and retained more rapidly and effectively than complex carbohydrates, as indicated by the NIH. Basic starches contain only a couple of sugars, for example, fructose (found in leafy foods) (found in milk items). These single sugars are called monosaccharides. Starch with two sugars —, for example, sucrose (table sugar), lactose (from dairy) and maltose (found in lager and a few vegetables) — are called disaccharides, as indicated by the NIH. Basic sugars are likewise in treat, pop and syrups. In any case, these nourishments are made with handled and refined sugars and don't have Vitamins, minerals or fiber. They are designated "void calories" and can prompt weight increase, as per the

NIH. Complex starches (polysaccharides) have at least three sugars. They are frequently alluded to as dull nourishments and incorporate beans, peas, lentils, peanuts, potatoes, corn, parsnips, entire grain breads and oats. Smathers called attention to that, while all starches work as moderately brisk vitality sources, basic carbohydrates cause explosions of vitality significantly more rapidly than complex sugars in view of the faster rate at which they are processed and ingested. Basic carbohydrates can prompt spikes in glucose levels and sugar rushes, while complex carbohydrates give increasingly supported vitality. Studies have indicated that supplanting saturated fats with straightforward carbohydrates, for example, those in many prepared nourishments, is related with an expanded danger of coronary illness and type 2 diabetes. Smathers offered the accompanying exhortation: "It's ideal to concentrate on getting essentially mind boggling carbohydrates in your eating routine, including entire grains and vegetables."

Sugars, Starches and Strands

In the body, carbohydrates separate into littler units of sugar, for example, glucose and fructose, as indicated by Iowa State University. The small digestive system retains these littler units, which at that point enter the circulation system and travel to the liver. The liver proselytes these sugars into glucose, which is helped through the circulation system — joined by insulin — and changed over into vitality for essential body working and physical action. In the event that the glucose isn't quickly required for vitality, the body can put away to 2,000 calories of it in the liver and skeletal muscles as glycogen, as indicated by Iowa State University. When glycogen stores are full, carbohydrates are put away as fat. In the event that you have lacking sugar admission or stores, the body will expend protein for fuel. This is risky in light of the fact that the body needs protein to make muscles. Utilizing protein rather than starches for fuel additionally puts weight on the kidneys, prompting the section of agonizing side-effects in the urine. Fiber is fundamental to absorption. Strands advance sound defecations and reduction the danger of interminable sicknesses, for example, coronary illness and diabetes, as indicated by the U.S. Division of Agriculture. Be that as it may, in contrast to sugars and starches, filaments are not caught up in the small digestive system and are not changed over to glucose. Rather, they go into the digestive organ generally flawless, where they are changed over to hydrogen and carbon dioxide and unsaturated fats. The Institute of Medicine suggests that individuals devour 14 grams of fiber for each 1,000 calories. sources of fiber incorporate organic products, grains and vegetables, particularly vegetables. Smathers brought up that carbohydrates are additionally found normally in certain types of dairy and both boring and nonstarchy vegetables. For instance, nonstarchy vegetables like lettuces, kale, green beans, celery, carrots and broccoli all contain carbohydrates. Boring vegetables like potatoes and corn additionally contain starches, however in bigger sums. As per the American Diabetes Association, nonstarchy vegetables for the most part contain just around 5 grams of starches for every cup of crude vegetables, and the vast majority of those carbohydrates originate from fiber.

Good carbohydrates versus bad carbohydrates

Sugars are found in nourishments you know are beneficial for you (vegetables) and ones you know are not (doughnuts). This has prompted the possibility that some carbohydrates are "great" and some are "awful." According to Healthy Geezer Fred Cicetti, carbohydrates generally thought to be awful incorporate baked goods, soft drinks, exceptionally prepared nourishments, a health doctor rice, a health doctor bread and other a health doctor-flour food sources. These are nourishments with basic carbohydrates. Terrible carbohydrates infrequently have any dietary benefit. Carbohydrates typically thought to be great are intricate carbohydrates, for example, entire grains, natural products, vegetables, beans and vegetables. These are prepared all the more gradually, however they additionally contain an abundance of different supplements.

The Pritikin Longevity Center offers this agenda for deciding whether a sugar is "good" or "bad"

Great carbohydrates are:

- Low or moderate in calories

- High in supplements

- Without refined sugars and refined grains

- High in normally happening fiber

- Low in sodium

- Low in soaked fat

- Exceptionally low in, or without, cholesterol

and trans fats

Bad carbohydrates are:

- High in calories

- Loaded with refined sugars, similar to corn syrup, a health doctor sugar, nectar and natural product juices

- High in refined grains like a health doctor flour

- Low in numerous supplements

- Low in fiber

- High in sodium

- Now and then high in soaked fat

- Now and then high in cholesterol and trans fats

Glycemic record

As of late, nutritionists have said that it's not the kind of sugar, yet rather the carb's glycemic file, that is significant. The glycemic record quantifies how rapidly and how much a starch raises glucose. High-glycemic nourishments like cakes raise glucose profoundly and quickly; low-glycemic food sources raise it tenderly and to a lesser degree. Some examination has connected high-glycemic nourishments with diabetes, heftiness, coronary illness and certain malignant growths, as indicated by Harvard Medical School. Then again, late research proposes that traceing a low-glycemic diet may not really be useful. A recent report distributed in JAMA found that overweight grown-ups eating a decent diet didn't see a lot of extra enhancement for a low-calorie, low-glycemic record diet. Researchers estimated insulin affectability, systolic circulatory strain, LDL cholesterol and HDL cholesterol and saw that the low-glycemic diet didn't improve them. It lowered triglycerides.

Benefits of Sugar

The correct sort of carbohydrates can be amazingly bravo. In addition to the fact that they are fundamental for your health, however they convey an assortment of included advantages.

Emotional Health

Sugars might be essential to emotional wellness. An examination distributed in 2009 in the diary JAMA

Internal Medicine found that individuals on a high-fat, low-carb diet for a year had more nervousness, wretchedness and outrage than individuals on a low-fat, high-carb diet. Researchers presume that sugars help with the generation of serotonin in the mind. Carbohydrates may support memory, as well. A recent report at Tufts University had overweight ladies cut carbohydrates altogether from their weight control plans for multi week. At that point, they tried the ladies' intellectual abilities, visual consideration and spatial memory. The ladies on no-carb counts calories did more regrettable than overweight ladies on low-calorie consumes less calories that contained a solid measure of starches.

Weight reduction

Despite the fact that carbohydrates are frequently accused for weight gain, the correct sort of carbohydrates can really assist you with losing and keep up a solid weight. This happens in light of the fact that numerous great starches, particularly entire grains and vegetable. What's most significant is the sort of starch you decide to eat on the grounds that a few sources are more advantageous than others. The measure of sugar in the eating routine – high or low – is less significant than the sort of starch in the eating regimen. For instance, solid, entire grains, for example, entire wheat bread, rye, grain and quinoa are preferable decisions over exceptionally refined a health doctor bread or French fries.Numerous individuals are confounded about starches, however remember that it's progressively essential to eat sugars from solid nourishments than to pursue a severe eating regimen constraining or tallying the quantity of grams of starches devoured.

What are starches?

Sugars are found in a wide exhibit of both solid and undesirable nourishments—bread, beans, milk, popcorn, potatoes, treats, spaghetti, sodas, corn, and cherry pie. They additionally arrive in an assortment of structures. The most widely recognized and bottomless structures are sugars, filaments, and starches. Nourishments high in sugars are a significant piece of a sound eating regimen. Sugars give the body glucose, which is changed over to vitality used to help substantial capacities and physical movement. However, sugar quality is significant; a few sorts of starch rich nourishments are superior to other people: The most beneficial sources of starches—natural or negligibly prepared entire grains, vegetables, foods grown from the ground—advance great health by conveying vitamins, minerals, fiber, and a large group of significant phytonutrients. Unhealthier sources of sugars incorporate a health doctor bread, baked goods, soft drinks, and other exceptionally prepared or refined nourishments. These things contain effectively processed sugars that may add to weight gain, meddle with weight reduction, and advance diabetes and coronary illness. The Healthy Eating Plate suggests filling a large portion of your plate with solid sugars – with vegetables (aside from potatoes) and natural products taking up about portion of your plate, and entire grains topping off around one fourth of your plate.

Attempt these tips for adding sound starches to your eating regimen:

- Start the day with entire grains.

Attempt a hot oat, similar to steel cut or antiquated oats (not moment oats), or a cool oat that rundowns an entire grain first on the fixing list and is low in sugar. A decent general guideline: Choose an oat that has at any rate 4 grams of fiber and under 8 grams of sugar for every serving.

- Utilize entire grain breads for lunch or tidbits.

Confounded about how to locate an entire grain bread? Search for bread that rundowns as the primary fixing entire wheat, entire rye, or some other entire grain — and stunningly better, one that is made with just entire grains, for example, 100 percent entire wheat bread.

• Likewise look past the bread path.

Entire wheat bread is regularly made with finely ground flour, and bread items are frequently high in sodium. Rather than bread, attempt an entire grain in plate of mixed greens structure, for example, dark colored rice or quinoa.

• Pick entire organic product rather than juice.

An orange has two fold the amount of fiber and half as much sugar as a 12-ounce glass of squeezed orange.

• Pass on potatoes, and rather expedite the beans.

Instead of top off on potatoes – which have been found to advance weight gain – pick beans for a magnificent source of gradually processed starches. Beans and different vegetables, for example, chickpeas additionally give a solid portion of protein.

CHAPTER FIVE

DIETARY FIBER

Dietary fiber is a starch that is not completely ingested in people and in certain creatures. Like all sugars, when it is processed it can deliver four Calories (kilocalories) of vitality per gram. In any case, much of the time it represents not as much as that as a result of its constrained ingestion and absorbability. Dietary fiber comprises primarily of cellulose, an enormous sugar polymer which is inedible as people don't have the necessary proteins to dismantle it. There are two subcategories: dissolvable and insoluble fiber. Entire grains, organic products (particularly plums, prunes, and figs), and vegetables are great sources of dietary fiber. There are numerous medical advantages of a high-fiber diet. Dietary fiber lessens the opportunity of gastrointestinal issues, for example, clogging and looseness of the bowels by expanding the weight and size of stool and relaxing it.

Insoluble fiber, found in entire wheat flour, nuts and vegetables, particularly animates peristalsis – the cadenced solid withdrawals of the digestive organs, which move digest along the stomach related tract. Solvent fiber, found in oats, peas, beans, and numerous organic products, breaks up in water in the intestinal tract to create a gel that eases back the development of nourishment through the digestion tracts. This may assist lower with blooding glucose levels since it can slow the ingestion of sugar. Also, fiber, maybe particularly that from entire grains, is thought to perhaps help diminish insulin spikes, and in this way lessen the danger of type 2 diabetes. The connection between expanded fiber utilization and a diminished danger of colorectal malignant growth is as yet dubious. Dietary fiber — found basically in natural products, vegetables, entire grains and vegetables — is likely most popular for its capacity to avoid or mitigate obstruction. Yet, nourishments containing fiber can give other medical advantages also, for example, keeping up a solid weight and bringing down your danger of diabetes, coronary illness and a few kinds of malignancy. Choosing delectable nourishments that give fiber isn't troublesome. Discover how much dietary fiber you need, the nourishments that contain it, and how to add them to dinners and bites. Fiber comprises for the most part of starches. Notwithstanding, in light of the fact that it isn't effectively consumed by the body, very little of the sugars and starches get into the circulation system. Fiber is a critical piece of sustenance, health, and fuel for gut microorganisms.

What is dietary fiber?

Dietary fiber, otherwise called roughage or mass, incorporates the pieces of plant nourishments your body can't process or assimilate. In contrast to other nourishment parts, for example, fats, proteins or sugars — which your body separates and assimilates — fiber isn't processed by your body. Rather, it goes generally unblemished through your stomach, small digestive tract and colon and out of your body. Dietary fiber is a kind of starch that can't be processed by our bodies' catalysts. It is found in palatable plant nourishments, for example, oats, natural products, vegetables, dried peas, nuts, lentils and grains. Fiber is assembled by its physical properties and is called solvent, insoluble or safe starch. Each of the three kinds of fiber have significant tasks to carry out. Dietary fiber helps keep the gut solid and is significant in lessening the danger of maladies, for example, diabetes, coronary illness and inside cancer2. Fiber arrives at the huge gut undigested where it is aged by microscopic organisms. The side-effects of this aging are carbon dioxide, methane, hydrogen and short-chain unsaturated fats (SCFAs). The SCFAs are utilized by the body. At first, expanding fiber admission can cause an expansion in gas creation which can bring about swelling. In any case, contingent upon the sort of fiber picked, our bodies do adjust and gas creation for a great many people should diminish after some time. Solvent fiber and safe starch likewise work as prebiotics and bolster the probiotics (microscopic organisms) we have in our enormous entrail which are fundamental for stomach related health. Fiber is generally named solvent, which breaks up in water, or insoluble, which doesn't disintegrate.

Soluble or Dissolvable fiber

This sort of fiber breaks down in water to frame a gel-like material. It can assist lower with blooding cholesterol and glucose levels. Solvent fiber is found in oats, peas, beans, apples, citrus natural products, carrots, grain and psyllium. Solvent fiber – which breaks down in water – is promptly matured in the colon into gases and physiologically dynamic side-effects, for example, short-chain unsaturated fats delivered in the colon by gut bacteria; it is gooey, might be called prebiotic fiber, and defers gastric discharging which, in people, can bring about an all-encompassing sentiment of fullness.

Insoluble fiber

This sort of fiber advances the development of material through your stomach related framework and expands stool mass, so it very well may be of advantage to the individuals who battle with stoppage or unpredictable stools. Entire wheat flour, wheat grain, nuts, beans and vegetables, for example, cauliflower, green beans and potatoes, are great sources of insoluble fiber. Insoluble fiber – which doesn't break up in water – is latent to stomach related chemicals in the upper gastrointestinal tract and gives bulking. Some types of insoluble fiber, for example, safe starches, can be aged in the colon. Bulking filaments ingest water as they travel through the stomach related framework, facilitating poo. The measure of dissolvable and insoluble fiber changes in various plant nourishments. To get the best medical advantage, eat a wide assortment of high-fiber nourishments.

Advantages of a High-fiber Diet

A high-fiber diet:

- ➤ Standardizes solid discharges: Dietary fiber builds the weight and size of your stool and relax it. A cumbersome stool is simpler to pass, diminishing your opportunity of stoppage. In the event that you have free, watery stools, fiber may cement the stool since it ingests water and adds mass to stool.

- ➤ Keeps up intestine health. A high-fiber diet may bring down your danger of creating hemorrhoids and little pockets in your colon (diverticular disease). Studies have likewise discovered that a high-fiber diet likely brings down the danger of colorectal malignant growth. Some fiber is matured in the colon. Specialists are taking a gander at how this may assume a job in anticipating infections of the colon.

- ➤ Brings down cholesterol levels. Solvent fiber found in beans, oats, flaxseed and oat wheat may assist lower with totaling blood cholesterol levels by bringing down low-thickness lipoprotein, or "terrible," cholesterol levels. Concentrates additionally have indicated that high-fiber nourishments may have other heart-medical advantages, for example, diminishing circulatory strain and aggravation.

➢ Assists control with blooding sugar levels. In individuals with diabetes, fiber — especially solvent fiber — can slow the ingestion of sugar and help improve glucose levels. A sound eating regimen that incorporates insoluble fiber may likewise decrease the danger of creating type 2 diabetes.

➢ Helps in accomplishing sound weight. High-fiber nourishments will in general be more filling than low-fiber nourishments, so you're probably going to eat less and remain fulfilled longer. What's more, high-fiber nourishments will in general take more time to eat and to be less "vitality thick," which implies they have less calories for a similar volume of nourishment.

➢ Encourages you live more. Studies recommend that expanding your dietary fiber consumption — particularly oat fiber — is related with a diminished danger of kicking the bucket from cardiovascular ailment and all diseases.

How much fiber do you need?

The Institute of Medicine, which gives science-put together guidance with respect to issues of medication and health, gives the accompanying every day fiber proposals for grown-ups:

Table 1. Fiber: Daily suggestions for grown-ups

	Age 50 or less	Age 50 or more
Men	38 grams	30 grams
Women	25 grams	21 grams

Your best fiber decisions

In the event that you aren't getting enough fiber every day, you may need to help your admission. Great decisions include:

- Entire grain items

- Organic products

- Vegetables

- Beans, peas and different vegetables

- Nuts and seeds

Refined or prepared nourishments —, for example, canned foods grown from the ground, mash free squeezes, a health doctor breads and pastas, and non-entire grain oats — are lower in fiber. The grain-refining process evacuates the external coat (wheat) from the grain, which brings down its fiber content. Enhanced nourishments have a portion of the B Vitamins and iron included back in the wake of preparing, however not the fiber.

Fiber supplements and sustained nourishments

Entire nourishments instead of fiber supplements are commonly better. Fiber supplements —, for example, Metamucil, Citrucel and FiberCon — don't give the assortment of filaments, Vitamins, minerals and other useful supplements that nourishments do. Another approach to get more fiber is to eat nourishments, for example, oat, granola bars, yogurt and dessert, with fiber included. The additional fiber as a rule is named as "inulin" or "chicory root." Some individuals gripe of gassiness subsequent to eating nourishments with included fiber. Be that as it may, a few people may at present need a fiber supplement if dietary changes aren't adequate or in the event that they have certain ailments, for example, blockage, the runs or touchy inside disorder. Check with your PCP before taking fiber supplements.

Tips for getting in more fiber

Need thoughts for adding more fiber to your suppers and tidbits? Attempt these proposals:

1) Kick off your day. For breakfast pick a high-fiber breakfast grain — at least 5 grams of fiber a serving. Settle on oats with "entire grain," "wheat" or "fiber" in the name. Or on the other hand include a couple of tablespoons of natural wheat grain to your preferred oat.

2) Change to entire grains. Devour at any rate half of all grains as entire grains. Search for breads that rundown entire wheat, entire wheat flour or another entire grain as the main fixing on the mark and have in any event 2 grams of dietary fiber a serving. Examination with dark colored rice, wild rice, grain, entire wheat pasta and bulgur wheat.

3) Beef up heated merchandise. Substitute entire grain flour for half or the entirety of the a health doctor flour when heating. Have a go at

including squashed grain oat, natural wheat grain or uncooked oats to biscuits, cakes and treats.

4) Incline toward vegetables. Beans, peas and lentils are brilliant sources of fiber. Add kidney beans to canned soup or a green serving of mixed greens. Or then again make nachos with refried dark beans, bunches of new veggies, entire wheat tortilla chips and salsa.

5) Eat more products of the soil. Products of the soil are plentiful in fiber, just as Vitamins and minerals. Attempt to eat at least five servings day by day.

6) Make the most of tidbits. Crisp organic products, crude vegetables, low-fat popcorn and entire grain wafers are on the whole great decisions. A bunch of nuts or dried natural products likewise is a solid, high-fiber nibble — in spite of the fact that know that nuts and dried organic products are high in calories.

7) High-fiber nourishments are useful for your health. However, including a lot of fiber also rapidly can advance intestinal gas, stomach

swelling and squeezing. Increment fiber in your eating regimen step by step over half a month. This permits the regular microscopic organisms in your stomach related framework to conform to the change.

8) Likewise, drink a lot of water. Fiber works best when it assimilates water, making your stool delicate and massive.

Where are the different types of fiber found?

Solvent fiber is found in nourishments like organic product, oats, beans and grain. At the point when it breaks down in water it shapes a gel-like substance. Dissolvable fiber serves to:

Bolster the development of neighborly microorganisms expected to help keep up a solid gut. It helps to also decrease cholesterol ingestion by official to it in the gut. Hinder the time it takes for nourishment to go through the stomach into the small digestive system This hinders the ingestion of glucose into the circulation system and has the advantages of keeping you feeling more full for more, controlling glucose levels, which are significant for the administration of diabetes. Safe Starch creates during the warming and afterward cooling of certain nourishments, for example, potato and rice. A few grains and grain items have been produced for their high safe starch levels and these incorporate Hi-maize and BARLEYmaxTM. Nourishments high in safe starch regularly have a low glycaemic record. Insoluble fiber doesn't break down in water and is found in nourishments like wholemeal bread, wheat grain, vegetables and nuts. Insoluble fiber adds mass to stools by engrossing water, and keeps you normal. It is critical to expand your liquid admission as you increment fiber. Without liquid, the fiber remains hard, making it hard to pass and causing clogging.

Which foods are rich in fiber?

Dietary fiber is found in natural products, vegetables, vegetables, wholegrain breads and grains. Most sources of dietary fiber will in general have a blend of both dissolvable and insoluble fiber in changing extents. Safe starch isn't constantly estimated when fiber is surveyed in a nourishment and we may think little of how much fiber is available in certain nourishments.

Nourishment Serving Size	Total Dietary Fiber (g)
Heated beans ½ cup	6.6
Untoasted Muesli 1 cup	2.7
Green peas ½ cup	3.4
Almond ½ cup	4.0
Wholemeal pasta 1 cup	8.4
Apple with skin 1 medium piece	2.3
Dried Apricots	4.5
Carrot, raw (120g)	4.0
Potato, cooked 1 medium (150g)	2.0
Multi grain bread	3.1

Recognize bundled nourishments that are sources of fiber, check the per serve segment of the sustenance data board. The business code of training uses the accompanying aide.

- Min 1.5g/serve = Source of fiber

- Min 3g/serve = High in fiber

- Min 6g/serve = Very high fiber

What amount do you need and is it possible to have too much?

By and large Australian grown-ups eat 18–25 g of fiber for each day and youngsters just 16g every day. Ongoing exploration proposes that over half of Australian grown-ups don't devour the prescribed 30 grams of fiber daily. 77% of the grown-ups that do meet the fiber consumption proposals have breakfast grain. Non breakfast grain eaters normal just somewhat more than 20 grams of fiber for every day. The nutrition types contributing most to day by day fiber admission were vegetables (30%), natural products (16%) and breakfast oats (12%). It has been recommended that accomplishing a fiber consumption higher than the normal can help lessen the danger of certain ailments. Presenting an excessive amount of fiber too rapidly or eating a lot of can cause clogging or looseness of the bowels in certain individuals. It is essential to bring fiber into your eating regimen step by step and guarantee that you drink satisfactory measures of liquid.

Tips for boosting fiber in yoir diet

It's anything but difficult to get more fiber in your eating regimen however recall, on the off chance that you're going from a low fiber diet, at that point include fiber in gradually and you won't endure the swelling inconvenience than can happen. Attempt a portion of these thoughts:

Change to a morning meal grain that is high in fiber; include some additional wheat, dried natural product or nuts. Porridge oats are likewise a decent decision as they contain solvent fiber Pick wholegrain or wholemeal bread rather than a health doctor. Change up sandwiches by including serving of mixed greens things, for example, lettuce, ground carrots and tomatoes

- Check evening desires by eating new natural product with the skin on as a tidbit

- Use wholegrain pasta rather than plain pasta when cooking your preferred pasta dish

- Build up stews by including new vegetables, grain, lentils and chickpeas

- Keep the skin on foods grown from the ground, as opposed to stripping them. Make sure to wash them well first.

- Top a heated potato with prepared beans, or put them in a toasted sandwich (Jaffle)

- Utilize dark colored rice instead of the more refined a health doctor rice. Most fiber is contained in the external layers of grains; the refining procedure expels these layers. Seeds and nuts can be a decent source of included fiber

Dietary fiber (British spelling fiber) or roughage is the segment of plant-inferred nourishment that can't be totally separated by human stomach related enzymes. It has two principle components: Dietary fiber comprises of non-starch polysaccharides and other plant parts, for example, cellulose, safe starch, safe dextrins, inulin, lignins, chitins, gelatins, beta-glucans, and oligosaccharides.Dietary strands can act by changing the idea of the substance of the gastrointestinal tract and by changing how different supplements and synthetic concoctions are absorbed. Some kinds of solvent fiber retain water to turn into a thick, gooey substance which might possibly be matured by microbes in the stomach related tract. A few sorts of insoluble fiber have building activity and are not fermented. Lignin, a significant dietary insoluble fiber source, may modify the rate and digestion of dissolvable fibers. Other kinds of insoluble fiber, quite safe starch, are matured to deliver short-chain unsaturated fats, which are physiologically dynamic and present health benefits. Health profit by dietary fiber and entire grains may incorporate a diminished danger of death and lower paces of coronary illness, colon malignant growth, and type 2 diabetes-Nourishment sources of dietary fiber have customarily been partitioned by whether they give dissolvable or insoluble fiber. Plant nourishments contain the two sorts of fiber in changing sums, as indicated by the plant's qualities of consistency and fermentability. Advantages of expending fiber rely on which kind of fiber is devoured and which advantages may result in the gastrointestinal system. Bulking strands –, for example, cellulose, hemicellulose and psyllium – retain and hold water, advancing regularity. Viscous filaments –, for example, beta-glucan and psyllium – thicken the fecal mass. Fermentable filaments –, for example, safe starch and inulin – feed the microscopic organisms and microbiota of the digestive organ, and are processed to yield short-chain unsaturated fats, which have different jobs in gastrointestinal health..

CHAPTER SIX

DIETARY FATS

A particle of dietary fat ordinarily comprises of a few unsaturated fats (containing long chains of carbon and hydrogen iotas), clung to a glycerol. They are commonly found as triglycerides (three unsaturated fats connected to one glycerol spine). Fats might be named soaked or unsaturated relying upon the point by point structure of the unsaturated fats included. Soaked fats have the entirety of the carbon iotas in their unsaturated fat chains clung to hydrogen particles, while unsaturated fats have a portion of these carbon iotas twofold reinforced, so their particles have generally less hydrogen molecules than an saturated unsaturated fat of a similar length. Unsaturated fats might be additionally delegated monounsaturated (one twofold security) or polyunsaturated (some twofold securities). Besides, contingent upon the area of the twofold security in the unsaturated fat chain, unsaturated fats are delegated omega-3 or omega-6 unsaturated fats. Trans fats are a kind of unsaturated fat with trans-isomer securities; these are uncommon in nature and in nourishments from characteristic sources; they are normally made in a modern procedure called (incomplete) hydrogenation. There are nine kilocalories in every gram of fat. Unsaturated fats, for example, conjugated linoleic corrosive, catalpic corrosive, eleostearic corrosive and punicic corrosive, notwithstanding giving vitality, speak to powerful resistant modulatory particles. Saturated fats (regularly from creature sources) have been a staple in numerous world societies for centuries. Unsaturated fats (e. g., vegetable oil) are viewed as more beneficial, while trans fats are to be stayed away from. saturated and some trans fats are ordinarily strong at room temperature, (for example, margarine or grease), while unsaturated fats are regularly fluids, (for example, olive oil or flaxseed oil). Trans fats are extremely uncommon in nature, and have been demonstrated to be exceptionally unfavorable to human health, however have properties helpful in the nourishment handling industry, for example, rancidity resistance.Oils and milk items are among the nourishments that contain fat. Despite the fact that it gets unfavorable criticism, fat is a significant supplement that the body needs so as to work. Eating the perfect sum — and the correct structure — of dietary fat is critical to keeping up great health, specialists state. Be that as it may, devouring a lot of fat or too little may mess health up. Fats are triglycerides - three particles of unsaturated fat joined with an atom of the liquor glycerol. Unsaturated fats are basic mixes (monomers) while triglycerides are mind boggling atoms (polymers). Fats are required in the eating regimen for health as they serve numerous capacities, including greasing up joints, helping organs produce hormones, aiding assimilation of specific Vitamins, decreasing irritation, and protecting mind health.

Capacity of fat

Fat is macronutrient. There are three macronutrients: protein, fats and sugars. Macronutrients are supplements that give calories or vitality. Huge sums are required to support life, consequently the expression "large scale," as per the University of Illinois McKinley Health Center. The measure of vitality gave by the macroVitamins shifts: fat has 9 calories for each gram, more than double the quantity of calories in carbohydrates and protein, which each have 4 calories for every gram. The essential capacity of fat is as a vitality hold, as indicated by Iowa State University. The body stores fat, or fat tissue, because of abundance calorie utilization. During exercise, the body first uses calories from starches for vitality. After around 20 minutes, it utilizes calories from put away fat to continue onward, as indicated by the National Institutes of Health (NIH). Fats additionally help the body ingest fundamental fat-dissolvable (Vitamins A, D, E and K), said Jim a health doctor, a Virginia Beach-based enlisted dietitian, health wellness authority and a representative for the Academy of Nutrition and Dietetics. Dietary fat likewise helps keep hair and skin solid, protects the body, secures organs and fills fat cells. "Fat assumes a job in the eating regimen and shouldn't be stayed away from," said a health doctor. "Your body needs sound sources of fat, otherwise called basic unsaturated fats, in light of the fact that the body can't deliver these unsaturated fats normally." Essential unsaturated fats add to mental health, blood coagulating and help in incendiary control, as indicated by the NIH.

Kinds of Fat

There are a few kinds of fat — some great, some awful, some surely knew and some less so. saturated fats and trans fats are usually viewed as undesirable, while unsaturated fats — including monounsaturated and polyunsaturated fat — are viewed as solid. All nourishments that contain fats have a blend of fat sorts, as per the Harvard School of Public Health.

Saturated Fats

Saturated fats are soaked with hydrogen atoms. As indicated by a health doctor, saturated fat originates from creature sources, for example, red meats, poultry and full-or-diminished fat dairy items. "Saturated fats are strong at room temperature," said Ximena Nutritionist, a Miami-based nutritionist and national representative for the Academy of Nutrition and Dietetics. She refered to grease for instance. Different models incorporate cheddar and spread. Oils that are strong at room temperature, similar to palm oil, palm bit oil and coconut oil, likewise contain saturated fats. This implies prepared merchandise can be high in soaked fats. "Saturated fat is connected to elevated cholesterol levels and an expanded danger of cardiovascular ailment," said a health doctor. Soaked fats additionally will in general contain a great deal of calories. The American Heart Association (AHA) prescribes getting just 5 to 6 percent of calories from saturated fat. This puts somebody on a 2,000-calorie-a-day diet with 120 calories or 13 grams of saturated fats every day. The 2010 U.S. Dietary Guidelines consider up to 10 percent of calories to originate from saturated fat.

Trans fats (additionally called trans

unsaturated fats)

As indicated by Nutritionist, trans fats are now and again found normally in meats or dairy, yet for the most part in limited quantities. All the more frequently, she stated, they are "delivered by the nourishment business for the reason to build time span of usability of the item." This is finished by adding hydrogen to fluid vegetable oils to make the oils increasingly strong. These are called mostly hydrogenated oils. Nutritionist said that they are frequently found in "advantageous nourishments" like solidified pizzas. Other basic sources of trans fats incorporate heated merchandise, saltines, refrigerated mixture, margarine and espresso half and half. Drive-through joints frequently use them in profound fryers in light of the fact that halfway hydrogenated oil doesn't need to be changed as regularly as customary oil. "Trans fats are not suggested at all in light of the connection to heart ailments," cautioned Nutritionist. Actually, they are regularly viewed as the most exceedingly awful kind of fat. As per the AHA, the two of them bring down your great cholesterol and increment your awful cholesterol. In 2013, the FDA proclaimed that incompletely hydrogenated oils were never again viewed as sheltered. There is as of now a three-year modification period set up with the goal that nourishment producers can change their practices or look for endorsement. Meanwhile, the Mayo Clinic prescribes checking names and searching for the words "mostly hydrogenated."

Triglycerides

Triglycerides are a possibly perilous kind of fat found in blood, as indicated by the NIH. They are related with coronary corridor ailment, particularly in ladies.

The body changes over any calories it doesn't have to utilize immediately into triglycerides, which are put away in the fat cells. They should give vitality between suppers, as indicated bya Research Center On the off chance that you eat a bigger number of calories than you use, in any case, the body doesn't consume triglycerides, and they collect. Most kinds of fat we eat become triglycerides. The Mayo Clinic gives the accompanying rules to solid triglyceride levels:

- Ordinary: Less than 150 milligrams for each deciliter (mg/dL), or under 1.7 millimoles per liter (mmol/L)

- Marginal high: 150 to 199 mg/dL (1.8 to 2.2 mmol/L)

- High: 200 to 499 mg/dL (2.3 to 5.6 mmol/L)

- Extremely High: 500 mg/dL or above (5.7 mmol/L or above)

A blood test can uncover your triglyceride levels.

Monounsaturated fats

These fats get their name since they are not saturated with hydrogen particles and on the grounds that they have a solitary carbon bond in the fat atom (called a twofold bond). "They are fluid at room temperature. Models are canola, nut or olive oil," said by a Nutritionist. Olives and avocadoes additionally contain monounsaturated fats, a health doctor included. "[Monounsaturated fats] are known to have a heart-defensive job," as said by a Nutritionist. a health doctor noticed that they have been connected to improved cholesterol levels, and the Mayo Clinic includes that they may help insulin levels and glucose control. It is as yet essential to watch your admission of monounsaturated fats in view of their high caloric substance, said Nutritionist. Despite the fact that there are no particular rules on what number of monounsaturated fats to devour, the Mayo Clinic recommends that the greater part of your all out fat admission should originate from sound fats.

Polyunsaturated fats

Like monounsaturated fats, polyunsaturated fats are not saturated with hydrogen particles. They get their name from having more than one carbon bond (twofold bond) in the fat particle, as indicated by the AHA. They are fluid at room temperature. Polyunsaturated fats are found generally in plant nourishment sources, for example, soybeans and soybean oil, sunflower oil, sunflower seeds, pecans and flaxseeds, a health doctor said. They're likewise present in fatty fish like salmon, fish, herring, mackerel and trout. "[Polyunsatured fats] have been appeared to affect blood cholesterol levels prompting a diminished danger of cardiovascular sickness," said a health doctor. They additionally help with cell improvement and upkeep and add Vitamin E to your eating regimen. Polyunsatured fats give basic unsaturated fats, including omega-6 and omega-3, as indicated by a health doctor. Despite the fact that there are no particular rules on what number of polyunsaturated fats to devour, the Mayo Clinic recommends that a large portion of your absolute fat admission should originate from solid fats.

Omega-3 unsaturated fats

"Omega-3 unsaturated fats are a polyunsaturated fat

that can emerge out of plant-based sources and are additionally found in fish," said a health doctor. "Omega-3 unsaturated fats have been appeared to bring down pulse levels." Nutritionists included that they are additionally significant enemy of inflammatories. On a cell level, omega-3 unsaturated fats work like headache medicine to restrain a catalyst that produces hormones that trigger irritation. They suggested eating cold-water fish like salmon, herring, fish and mackerel, just as pecans, olive oil and canola oil. A few people take fish oil to up their omega-3 admission. There are no standard proposals for the measure of omega-3s you need each day. The American Heart Association suggests eating 3.5 ounces of fish at any rate two times every week to get a decent measure of omega-3s. Nobody ought to expend multiple grams of omega-3s from supplements without counseling a specialist, as it might cause dying.

Omega-6 unsaturated fats

"Omega-6 unsaturated fats are additionally polyunsaturated fats generally found in plant-based oils," said a health doctor. Great sources incorporate vegetable, corn, nut, grapeseed and sunflower oils, just as mayonnaise and numerous plate of mixed greens dressings. As indicated by a health doctor, omega-6 unsaturated fats advance solid skin and hair development and advantage a sound digestion. They likewise help keep up bone health and the regenerative framework. In unnecessary sums, a few kinds of solid omega-6 unsaturated fats may make the body produce fiery synthetic substances, as indicated by the University of Maryland Medical Center. This is critical to note in light of the fact that when all is said in done, Americans get definitely more omega-6 unsaturated fats than should be expected and extremely not many omega-3s. The American Heart Association prescribes that somewhere in the range of 5 and 10 percent of calories originate from omega-6 unsaturated fats.

Finding the balance

Your fat utilization ought to be relative to your weight and dietary way of life," said a health doctor. In case you're attempting to change your body or get more beneficial, it ought to be corresponding to your objectives. "You should take a gander at what number of calories you have to expend day by day to keep up, get more fit, or put on weight (in view of your objectives)." A health doctor said that the normal grown-up ought to get 20 to 35 percent of their calories from sound fat sources. A grown-up eating a 2,000-calorie-a-day diet could eat 44 to 78 grams of fat in a day. Some solid fat sources incorporate olive oil, avocadoes, salmon, fish, pecans, flax seeds and sunflower seeds, said by the health doctor. "Emotional well-being shortfalls like gloom and lack of vitamins can happen. The Vitamins A, D, E and K are fat dissolvable, which means the body stores them in fatty tissue and the liver. The digestion tracts need dietary fat to appropriately assimilate these supplements. These Vitamins are likewise essential for the health of your skin, bones and cardiovascular framework, among different organs and frameworks."

"It isn't normal for somebody to be insufficient in fat in their eating routine, the vast majority are blameworthy of having an excess of fat in their eating regimen. Anything over a normal sum is excessively," said a health doctor. In the event that you eat an excess of fat, you will probably put on weight, which is connected to medical issues. Research on fat is progressing, yet a few examinations recommend that abundance fat may assume a job in coronary illness, malignant growth and type 2 diabetes, as indicated by a Research Center Eating an excessive amount of fat is additionally connected to elevated cholesterol.

Changing dietary rules for fat

At regular intervals, the U.S. Branch of Agriculture (USDA) and the U.S. Division of Health and Human Services (HHS) make an advisory group to refresh the authority U.S. Dietary Guidelines. The most present variant accessible is from 2010. That variant informs that 20 to 35 percent regarding calories originate from fat. In 2015, notwithstanding, the Dietary Guidelines Advisory Committee (DGAC) gave a proposal to expel limitations on fat utilization. There is a developing group of proof that underlines getting solid fats and keeping away from unfortunate ones instead of cutting fats by and large, as pera Research Center a health doctor encourages not to cut all dietary fat, however to monitor it. "Concentrate on devouring solid fat sources rather than unfortunate fat to help toward weight reduction objectives," he said. Besides, low-fat eating regimens regularly lead to individuals eating profoundly prepared nourishments that are high in refined sugar and starches however low in fat. As opposed to indicating how much fat to expend, the DGAC exhorted eating more vegetables and restricting sugar. As of this composition, the 2015 Dietary Guidelines had not been distributed so it is obscure if the USDA and HHS took the suggestion.

Basic fatty acids

Most unsaturated fats are insignificant, which means the body can deliver them as required, for the most part from other unsaturated fats and consistently by using vitality to do as such. Be that as it may, in people, in any event two unsaturated fats are fundamental and must be remembered for the eating routine. A fitting parity of fundamental unsaturated fats—omega-3 and omega-6 unsaturated fats—appears to be likewise significant for health, albeit authoritative test show has been tricky. Both of these "omega" long-chain polyunsaturated unsaturated fats are substrates for a class of eicosanoids known as prostaglandins, which have jobs all through the human body. They are hormones, in certain regards. The omega-3 eicosapentaenoic corrosive (EPA), which can be made in the human body from the omega-3 basic unsaturated fat alpha-linolenic corrosive (ALA), or taken in through marine nourishment sources, fills in as a structure hinder for arrangement 3 prostaglandins (e.g., feebly incendiary PGE3). The omega-6 dihomo-gamma-linolenic corrosive (DGLA) fills in as a structure obstruct for arrangement 1 prostaglandins (for example mitigating PGE1), while arachidonic corrosive (AA) fills in as a structure hinder for arrangement 2 prostaglandins (for example master incendiary PGE

2). Both DGLA and AA can be produced using the omega-6 linoleic corrosive (LA) in the human body, or can be taken in straightforwardly through nourishment. A properly adjusted admission of omega-3 and omega-6 somewhat decides the general creation of various prostaglandins, which is one motivation behind why a harmony between omega-3 and omega-6 is accepted significant for cardiovascular health. In industrialized social orders, individuals commonly expend a lot of handled vegetable oils, which have decreased measures of the basic unsaturated fats alongside a lot of omega-6 unsaturated fats comparative with omega-3 unsaturated fats. The transformation pace of omega-6 DGLA to AA to a great extent decides the creation of the prostaglandins PGE1 and PGE2. Omega-3 EPA keeps AA from being discharged from layers, in this way slanting prostaglandin balance away from professional incendiary PGE2 (produced using AA) toward mitigating PGE1 (produced using DGLA). Also, the transformation (desaturation) of DGLA to AA is constrained by the protein delta-5-desaturase, which thusly is constrained by hormones, for example, insulin (up-guideline) and glucagon (down-guideline). The sum and kind of sugars devoured, alongside certain sorts of amino corrosive, can impact forms including insulin, glucagon, and different hormones; consequently, the proportion of omega-3 versus omega-6 effectsly affects general health, and explicit consequences for resistant capacity and aggravation, and mitosis (i.e., cell division). These days, we are shelled with wellness online journals, Instagram posts, and Facebook notices that toss around the term macros. Macros is the shortened form for macroVitamins. In any case, what are macroVitamins, for what reason would they say they are so well known in the wellness and nourishment world, and what proportion is perfect for you? Our nutritionists will clarify. One of the primary issues with conventional eating less junk food is that calorie checking doesn't consider what you're eating. Macros can be a key player here, helping us measure the amount we eat just as what we eat. Considering macros rather than calories — something 8fit feast plans fare thee well — helps move you into a more advantageous, all the more balanced method for eating.

CHAPTER SEVEN

PROTEINS

Proteins are auxiliary materials in a significant part of the creature body (for example muscles, skin, and hair). They likewise structure the proteins that control concoction responses all through the body. Every protein particle is made out of amino acids, which are described by incorporation of nitrogen and once in a while sulfur (these segments are answerable for the unmistakable smell of consuming protein, for example, the keratin in hair). The body requires amino acids to create new proteins (protein maintenance) and to supplant harmed proteins (support). As there is no protein or amino corrosive stockpiling arrangement, amino acids must be available in the eating regimen. Abundance amino acids are disposed of, commonly in the urine. For all creatures, some amino acids are fundamental (a creature can't deliver them inside) and some are superfluous (the creature can create them from other nitrogen-containing mixes). Around twenty amino acids are found in the human body, and around ten of these are basic and, accordingly, must be remembered for the eating regimen. An eating regimen that contains sufficient measures of amino acids (particularly those that are fundamental) is especially significant in certain circumstances: during early improvement and development, pregnancy, lactation, or damage (a consume, for example). A total protein source contains all the fundamental amino acids; a fragmented protein source needs at least one of the basic amino acids. It is conceivable with protein mixes of two fragmented protein sources (e.g., rice and beans) to make a total protein source, and trademark mixes are the premise of unmistakable social cooking conventions. Be that as it may, reciprocal sources of protein don't should be eaten at a similar dinner to be utilized together by the body. Excess amino acids from protein can be changed over into glucose and utilized for fuel through a procedure called gluconeogenesis

. Proteins are fundamental supplements for the human body. They are one of the structure squares of body tissue and can likewise fill in as a fuel source. As a fuel, proteins give as a lot of vitality thickness as starches: 4 kcal (17 kJ) per gram; conversely, lipids give 9 kcal (37 kJ) per gram. The most significant viewpoint and characterizing normal for protein from a dietary stance is its amino corrosive composition. Proteins are polymer chains made of amino acids connected together by peptide bonds. During human absorption, proteins are separated in the stomach to littler polypeptide chains through hydrochloric corrosive and protease activities. This is vital for the ingestion of the fundamental amino acids that can't be biosynthesized by the body. There are nine basic amino acids which people must acquire from their eating regimen so as to avert protein-vitality unhealthiness and coming about death. They are phenylalanine, valine, threonine, tryptophan, methionine, leucine, isoleucine, lysine, and histidine. There has been banter with respect to whether there are 8 or 9 fundamental amino acids. The accord appears to fit towards 9 since histidine isn't combined in adults. There are five amino acids which people can incorporate in the body. These five are alanine, aspartic corrosive, asparagine, glutamic corrosive and serine. There are six restrictively fundamental amino acids whose amalgamation can be constrained under uncommon pathophysiological conditions, for example, rashness in the newborn child or people in serious catabolic pain. These six are arginine, cysteine, glycine, glutamine, proline and tyrosine. Every single dietary source of protein incorporate the two creatures and plants: meats, dairy items, fish and eggs, just as grains, vegetables and nuts. Veggie lovers can get enough fundamental amino acids by eating plant proteins like beans and nuts. Protein can be found in a wide scope of nourishment. The best blend of protein sources relies upon the locale of the world, get to, cost, amino corrosive sorts and nourishment balance, just as procured tastes. A few nourishments are high in certain amino acids, however their edibility and the counter healthful components present in these food sources make them of constrained an incentive in human sustenance. In this manner, one must consider absorbability and auxiliary sustenance profile, for example, calories, cholesterol, Vitamins and basic mineral thickness of the protein source. On an overall premise, plant protein nourishments contribute more than 60 percent of the per capita supply of protein, by and large. In North America, creature inferred nourishments contribute around 70 percent of protein sources.Meat, items from milk, eggs, soy, and fish are sources of complete protein. Entire grains and oats are another source of proteins. Be that as it may, these will in general be constraining in the amino corrosive lysine or threonine, which are accessible in other vegan sources and meats. Instances of nourishment staples and grain sources of protein, each with a fixation more noteworthy than

7.0%, are (in no specific request) buckwheat, oats, rye, millet, maize (corn), rice, wheat, sorghum, amaranth, and quinoa. Veggie lover sources of proteins incorporate vegetables, nuts, seeds and natural products. Vegetables, some of which are called beats in specific pieces of the world, have higher groupings of amino acids and are more finished sources of protein than entire grains and oats. Instances of veggie lover nourishments with protein fixations more prominent than 7 percent incorporate soybeans, lentils, kidney beans, a health doctor beans, mung beans, chickpeas, cowpeas, lima beans, pigeon peas, lupines, wing beans, almonds, Brazil nuts, cashews, walnuts, pecans, cotton seeds, pumpkin seeds, hemp seeds, sesame seeds, and sunflower seeds.

Plant sources of protein.

Nourishment supply from plants are poor sources of protein; it incorporate roots and tubers, for example, yams, cassava and sweet potato. Plantains, another significant staple, are additionally a poor source of fundamental amino acids. Natural products, while wealthy in other fundamental supplements, are another poor source of amino acids. The protein content in roots, tubers and organic products is somewhere in the range of 0 and 2 percent. Nourishment staples with low protein content must be supplemented with food sources with complete, quality protein content for a solid life, especially in kids for legitimate development. A decent source of protein is regularly a blend of different nourishments, on the grounds that various food sources are wealthy in various amino acids. A decent source of dietary protein meets two requirements: The prerequisite for the healthfully essential amino acids (histidine, isoleucine, leucine, lysine, methionine, phenylalanine, threonine, tryptophan, and valine) under all conditions and for restrictively basic amino acids (cystine, tyrosine, taurine, glycine, arginine, glutamine, proline) under explicit physiological and neurotic conditions The necessity for vague nitrogen for the combination of the healthfully unnecessary amino acids (aspartic corrosive, asparagine, glutamic corrosive, alanine, serine) and other physiologically significant nitrogen-containing mixes, for example, nucleic acids, creatine, and porphyrins.

Sound individuals eating a fair diet seldom need protein supplements.

Significant discussion has occurred with respect to issues encompassing protein admission requirements. The measure of protein required in an individual's eating regimen is resolved in enormous part by in general vitality consumption, the body's requirement for nitrogen and basic amino acids, body weight and sythesis, pace of development in the individual, physical action level, the person's vitality and sugar admission, and the nearness of ailment or injury. Physical movement and effort just as upgraded strong mass increment the requirement for protein. Prerequisites are additionally more prominent during adolescence for development and advancement, during pregnancy, or while breastfeeding so as to sustain an infant or when the body needs to recuperate from lack of healthy sustenance or injury or after an operation. If insufficient vitality is taken in through diet, as during the time spent starvation, the body will utilize protein from the bulk to meet its vitality needs, prompting muscle burning through after some time. In the event that the individual doesn't devour sufficient protein in nourishment, at that point muscle will likewise squander as increasingly indispensable cell forms (e.g., breath catalysts, platelets) reuse muscle protein for their very own requirements.[citation needed]

Dietary recommendations

As per US and Canadian Dietary Reference Intake rules, ladies matured 19–70 need to devour 46 grams of protein for every day while men matured 19–70 need to expend 56 grams of protein for every day to limit danger of lack. These Recommended Dietary Allowances (RDAs) were determined dependent on 0.8 grams protein per kilogram body weight and normal body loads of 57 kg (126 pounds) and 70 kg (154 pounds), respectively. However, this suggestion depends on auxiliary necessities yet ignores utilization of protein for vitality metabolism. This prerequisite is for a typical stationary person. In the United States, normal protein utilization is higher than the RDA. As indicated by aftereffects of the National Health and Nutrition Examination Survey (NHANES 2013-2014), normal protein utilization for ladies ages 20 and more established was 69.8 grams and for men 98.3 grams/day.

Dynamic people

A few examinations have reasoned that dynamic individuals and competitors may require raised protein consumption (contrasted with 0.8 g/kg) because of increment in bulk and sweat misfortunes, just as requirement for body fix and vitality source. Suggested sums differ from 1.2-1.4 g/kg for those doing continuance exercise to as much as 1.6-1.8 g/kg for quality exercise, while a proposed greatest day by day protein admission would be around 25% of vitality prerequisites for example roughly 2 to 2.5 g/kg. However, numerous inquiries still stay to be resolved. Furthermore, some have recommended that competitors utilizing limited calorie eats less carbohydrates for weight reduction should additionally expand their protein utilization, perhaps to 1.8–2.0 g/kg, so as to stay away from loss of slender muscle mass.

Vigorous exercise protein needs

Continuance competitors contrast from quality structure competitors in that perseverance competitors don't work as a lot of bulk from preparing as quality structure competitors do. [citation needed] Research recommends that people performing perseverance action require more protein admission than stationary people so muscles separated during continuance exercises can be repaired. Although the protein prerequisite for competitors still stays questionable (for example observe Lamont, Nutrition Research Reviews, pages 142 - 149, 2012), inquire about shows that perseverance competitors can profit by expanding protein consumption in light of the fact that the sort of activity continuance competitors take an interest in still modifies the protein digestion pathway. The general protein necessity builds due to amino corrosive oxidation in continuance prepared athletes. Endurance competitors who practice over a significant stretch (2–5 hours for every instructional meeting) use protein as a source of 5–10% of their all out vitality used. In this manner, a slight increment in protein admission might be advantageous to perseverance competitors by supplanting the protein lost in vitality consumption and protein lost in fixing muscles. One audit reasoned that perseverance competitors may expand every day protein admission to a limit of 1.2–1.4 g per kg body weight.

Anaerobic exercise protein needs

Research likewise demonstrates that people performing quality preparing action require more protein than stationary people. Quality preparing competitors may expand their every day protein admission to a limit of 1.4–1.8 g per kg body weight to improve muscle protein combination, or to compensate for the loss of amino corrosive oxidation during exercise. Numerous competitors keep up a high-protein diet as a component of their preparation. Indeed, a few competitors who have practical experience in anaerobic games (e.g., weightlifting) accept an exceptionally elevated level of protein admission is vital, thus devour high protein dinners and furthermore protein supplements.

Protein allergies   or disorders

A nourishment sensitivity is a strange safe reaction to proteins in nourishment. The signs and manifestations may go from gentle to extreme. They may incorporate irritation, expanding of the tongue, heaving, looseness of the bowels, hives, inconvenience breathing, or low circulatory strain. These side effects commonly happens inside minutes to one hour after presentation. At the point when the side effects are serious, it is known as hypersensitivity. The accompanying eight nourishments are answerable for about 90% of unfavorably susceptible responses: dairy animals' milk, eggs, wheat, shellfish, fish, peanuts, tree nuts and soy.

Constant kidney disease

While there is no decisive proof that a high protein diet can cause constant kidney ailment, there is an accord that individuals with this sickness should diminish utilization of protein. As indicated by one 2009 audit, individuals with incessant kidney sickness who diminish protein utilization have a 32% lower danger of death in contrast with influenced individuals who don't make these dietary changes. [38][needs update][39] Moreover, individuals with this infection while utilizing a low protein diet (0.6 g/kg/d - 0.8 g/kg/d) may create metabolic remunerations that protect kidney work, in spite of the fact that in certain individuals, lack of healthy sustenance may occur.

Phenylketonuria

People with phenylketonuria (PKU) must keep their admission of phenylalanine - a fundamental amino corrosive - very low to avoid a psychological incapacity and other metabolic entanglements. Phenylalanine is a segment of the fake sugar aspartame, so individuals with PKU need to evade low calorie refreshments and nourishments with this ingredient.

Maple syrup urine disease

Maple syrup urine illness is related with hereditary peculiarities in the digestion of stretched chain amino acids (BCAAs). They have high blood levels of BCAAs and should seriously confine their admission of BCAAs so as to counteract mental impediment and passing. The amino acids being referred to are leucine, isoleucine and valine. The condition gets its name from the unmistakable sweet smell of influenced newborn children's urine. Offspring of Amish, Mennonite, and Ashkenazi Jewish plummet have a high predominance of this illness contrasted with other populations. Protein lack and ailing health (PEM) can prompt assortment of sicknesses including mental hindrance and kwashiorkor. Symptoms of kwashiorkor incorporate disregard, loose bowels, dormancy, inability to develop, flaky skin, fatty liver, and edema of the paunch and legs. This edema is clarified by the activity of lipoxygenase on arachidonic corrosive to frame leukotrienes and the ordinary working of proteins in liquid parity and lipoprotein transport. PEM is genuinely regular worldwide in the two kids and grown-ups and represents 6 million passings every year. In the industrialized world, PEM is overwhelmingly found in clinics, is related with disease, or is frequently found in the elderly.

CHAPTER EIGHT

WATER

Water is discharged from the body in various structures; including urine and dung, perspiring, and by water fume in the breathed out breath. Along these lines, it is important to enough rehydrate to supplant lost liquids. Early proposals for the amount of water required for support of good health proposed that 6–8 glasses of water day by day is the base to keep up legitimate hydration. However the thought that an individual ought to expend eight glasses of water for each day can't be traceed to a valid logical source. The first water consumption suggestion in 1945 by the Food and Nutrition Board of the National Research Council read: "A normal standard for differing people is 1 milliliter for every calorie of nourishment. The greater part of this amount is contained in arranged foods." More ongoing examinations of surely understood proposals on liquid admission have uncovered enormous inconsistencies in the volumes of water we have to expend for good health. Therefore, to help institutionalize rules, suggestions for water utilization are remembered for two latc European Food Safety Authority (EFSA) archives (2010): (I) Food-based dietary rules and (ii) Dietary reference esteems for water or sufficient every day admissions (ADI). These details were given by ascertaining satisfactory admissions from estimated admissions in populaces of people with "attractive osmolarity estimations of urine and alluring water volumes per vitality unit consumed." For empowering hydration, the flow EFSA rules prescribe all out water admissions of 2.0 L/day for grown-up females and 2.5 L/day for grown-up guys. These reference esteems incorporate water from drinking water, different refreshments, and from nourishment. About 80% of our day by day water prerequisite originates from the refreshments we drink, with the staying 20% originating from food. Water content differs relying upon the kind of nourishment expended, with leafy foods containing more than oats, for example.[68]. These qualities are evaluated utilizing nation explicit nourishment monetary records distributed by the Food and Agriculture Organization of the United Nations.The EFSA board additionally decided admissions for various populaces. Prescribed admission volumes in the old are equivalent to for grown-ups as regardless of lower vitality utilization, the water necessity of this gathering is expanded because of a decrease in renal concentrating capacity. Pregnant and breastfeeding ladies require extra liquids to remain hydrated. The EFSA board suggests that pregnant ladies ought to devour a similar volume of water as non-pregnant ladies, in addition to an expansion in relation to the higher vitality necessity, equivalent to 300 mL/day. To make up for extra liquid yield, breastfeeding ladies require an extra 700 mL/day over the prescribed admission esteems for non-lactating ladies. Drying out and over-hydration - excessively little and a lot of water, individually - can have hurtful results. Drinking an excessive amount of water is one of the potential reasons for hyponatremia, i.e., low serum sodium. Health specialists state that water is a fundamental supplement and prescribe drinking a lot of it. The dietary benefit of water doesn't appear to be excessively great, however. What you can be sure of is that its piece relies upon the source. Sufficient water admission is imperative for good sustenance.

For what reason Do You Need Water?

Water makes up 50 to 75 percent of the human body. It's an indispensable segment of your blood, salivation, stomach related juices, cells and tissues. It saturates your skin, greases up your joints, conveys oxygen to your cells and assists flush with trip squander, among different capacities. This crucial liquid is likewise vital for vitality digestion. It disintegrates minerals, water-dissolvable Vitamins and different supplements with the goal that your body can utilize them. Besides, water directs your internal heat level and guarantees appropriate processing. It additionally encourages you keep up a solid weight and keeps you hydrated. Around 70 percent of the non-fat mass of the human body is water. It is indispensable for some procedures in the human body. No one is totally certain how much water the human body needs - claims differ from 1-7 liters for every day to dodge lack of hydration. We do realize that water necessities are firmly connected to body size, age, natural temperatures, physical action, various conditions of health, and dietary propensities; for example, someone who expends a great deal of salt will require more water than another comparable individual. Cases that 'the more water you drink, the more advantageous you are' are not sponsored with logical proof. The factors that impact water prerequisites are tremendous to such an extent that exact guidance on water admission would just be substantial in the wake of assessing every individual exclusively. As per a smaller than normal survey distributed in the June 2016 release of Frontiers in Nutrition, expanded hydration may encourage weight reduction and ensure against diabetes. Specialists state that water may help avoid weight because of its thermogenic properties. Furthermore, it might animate lipolysis, or fat breakdown, and hoist your digestion. In addition, you don't need to stress over water calories. Simply ensure you avoid enhanced water, Vitamin water and other sugary refreshments. Plain water has no additional sugar, calories, added substances or additives. It extinguishes your thirst and tops you off rapidly, which thusly, may help counteract gorging.

Water Nutrition Facts

Water contains no protein, carbohydrates or fats, so does it have any dietary benefit? The appropriate response is yes. A wide range of water, including faucet water, give trace components, for example, copper, magnesium and chloride. Springwater and shining mineral water are the most out of this world, from underground sources plentiful in minerals and trace components. Here's a fast breakdown of the various kinds of water, per one-cup serving:

- Faucet water — 7 mg of calcium, 2 mg of magnesium, 9 mg of sodium and 0.02 mg of zinc

- Common shimmering mineral water — 60 mg of calcium and 17 mg of magnesium

- Evian water — 19 mg of calcium and 5 mg of magnesium

- Perrier water — 33 mg of calcium and 2 mg of sodium

- Conventional filtered water — 24 mg of calcium, 5 mg of magnesium and 5 mg of sodium

Calcium, one of the trace minerals in water, keeps your bones and teeth sound, directs heartbeat and adds to blood coagulating. The day by day prescribed admission for grown-ups is 1,000 milligrams, as per the U.S. National Library of Medicine. Characteristic shining mineral water, for instance, gives 60 milligrams of calcium for every cup. On the off chance that you drink eight cups per day, that is 480 milligrams of calcium — practically 50% of the day by day suggested consumption. Water is likewise a decent source of magnesium. This mineral controls vitality digestion, glucose levels, heartbeat, muscle compressions and that's only the tip of the iceberg. The prescribed every day recompense is 400 to 420 milligrams for grown-up men and 310 to 320 milligrams for grown-up ladies. Most kinds of filtered water have around 5 milligrams of magnesium for each cup, so eight cups will give 40 milligrams of this supplement. That is around 10 percent of the day by day suggested magnesium admission for men.

Does Water Promote Weight Loss?

This zero-calorie refreshment can make it simpler to get more fit. It expands satiety as well as lessens your all out nourishment admission and lifts your digestion. An associate report distributed in the diary Vitamins in October 2016 recommends that supplanting one serving of pop or brew every day with water may forestall stoutness and encourage weight reduction. Heftiness is a significant hazard factor for diabetes, coronary illness and other constant diseases, so water utilization may secure against these afflictions by helping you accomplish a typical weight. In case you're constantly eager or wanting to nibble, taste on carbonated water. This drink may improve hunger control and increment satiety, as indicated by a little report included in the Journal of Nutritional Science and Vitaminology in February 2012. Female subjects who drank carbonated water experienced more prominent satiety than those drinking plain water. Recollect that water has no calories. Use it as a substitute for caffeinated drinks, coke, cappuccino, frappe, milkshakes and other sugary refreshments. This little change can assist you with sparing two or three hundred calories every day. It takes a 3,500-calorie shortfall to lose one pound of fat, implying that you can get less fatty inside weeks just by swapping soft drink for plain water.

Alcohol (ethanol) Unadulterated ethanol gives 7 calories for each gram. For refined spirits, a standard serving in the United States is 1.5 liquid ounces, which at 40% ethanol (80 proof), would be 14 grams and 98 calories. Wine and brew contain a comparable scope of ethanol for servings of 5 ounces and 12 ounces, separately, however these refreshments additionally contain non-ethanol calories. A 5 ounce serving of wine contains 100 to 130 calories. A 12 ounce serving of brew contains 95 to 200 calories. According to the U.S. Division of Agriculture, in light of NHANES 2013-2014 studies, ladies ages 20 and up devour all things considered 6.8 grams/day and men expend overall 15.5 grams/day. Ignoring the non-liquor commitment of those refreshments, the normal ethanol calorie commitments are 48 and 108 cal/day. Mixed refreshments are viewed as vacant calorie nourishments in light of the fact that other than calories, these contribute no fundamental supplements.

CHAPTER NINE

MICRONUTRIENTS

Micronutrients are basic components required by living beings in changing amounts all through life to organize a scope of physiological capacities to keep up health. Micronutrient prerequisites vary between creatures; for instance, people and different creatures require various Vitamins and dietary minerals, while plants require explicit minerals. For human nourishment, micronutrients necessities are in sums commonly under 100 milligrams for each day, though macroVitamins are required in gram amounts day by day.

Called micronutrients since they are required uniquely in little sums, these substances are the "enchantment wands" that empower the body to deliver catalysts, hormones and different substances fundamental for appropriate development and advancement. As minor as the sums seem to be, be that as it may, the outcomes of their nonappearance are serious. Iodine, nutrient An and iron are generally significant in worldwide general wellbeing terms; their need speaks to a significant danger to the wellbeing and improvement of populaces the world over, especially youngsters and pregnant ladies in low-pay nations. The minerals for people and different creatures incorporate 13 components that begin from Earth's dirt and are not blended by living beings, for example, calcium and iron. Micronutrients are necessities for creatures additionally incorporate Vitamins, which are natural mixes required in microgram or milligram amounts. Since plants are the essential starting point of supplements for people and creatures, a few micronutrient might be in low levels and lacks can happen when dietary admission is deficient, as happens in unhealthiness, suggesting the requirement for activities to dissuade insufficient microVitamin supply in plant foods

Micronutrients: Types, Functions, Benefits and the sky is the limit from there

Micronutrients are one of the significant gatherings of supplements your body needs. They incorporate Vitamins and minerals. Vitamins are fundamental for vitality creation, insusceptible capacity, blood coagulating and different capacities. In the interim, minerals assume a significant job in development, bone health, liquid parity and a few different procedures. This chapter gives a definite review of micronutrients, their capacities and ramifications of overabundance utilization or inadequacy.

What Are Micronutrients?

The term micronutrients is utilized to portray Vitamins and minerals as a rule. Macronutrients, then again, incorporate proteins, fats and starches. Your body needs littler measures of micronutrients comparative with macroVitamins. That is the reason they're named "small scale." People must get micronutrients from nourishment since your body can't deliver Vitamins and minerals — generally. That is the reason they're likewise alluded to as fundamental supplements. Vitamins are natural mixes made by plants and creatures which can be separated by warmth, corrosive or air. Then again, minerals are inorganic, exist in soil or water and can't be separated. At the point when you eat, you devour the Vitamins that plants and creatures made or the minerals they assimilated. The micronutrients substance of every nourishment is unique, so it's ideal to eat an assortment of food sources to get enough Vitamins and minerals. A sufficient admission of all micronutrient is vital for ideal health, as every Vitamin and mineral has a particular job in your body. Vitamins and minerals are fundamental for development, invulnerable capacity, mental health and numerous other significant capacities. Contingent upon their capacity, certain micronutrient additionally assume a job in forestalling and battling disease. Micronutrients incorporate Vitamins and minerals. They're basic for a few significant capacities in your body and should be expended from nourishment.

Types and Functions of Micronutrients

Vitamins and minerals can be separated into four classifications: water-solvent Vitamins, fat-dissolvable Vitamins, macrominerals and trace minerals. Notwithstanding type, Vitamins and minerals are caught up in comparative manners in your body and cooperate in numerous procedures. Various micronutrients powder of at any rate iron, zinc, and Vitamin A was added to the World Health Organization's List of Essential Medicines in 2019

The micronutrients are minerals, vitamins, and others.

Micronutrients – otherwise called nutrients and minerals – are fundamental parts of a top notch eat less carbs and profoundly affect wellbeing. While they are just required in modest amounts, micronutrients are the basic structure squares of sound minds, bones and bodies. Expending a various scope of supplement thick nourishments close by breastfeeding is the perfect path for small kids to get basic micronutrients in their eating regimens. Yet, in numerous pieces of the world, youngsters' weight control plans contain inadequate micronutrients and insufficiencies are far reaching. Micronutrient inadequacies are frequently alluded to as 'shrouded hunger' since they grow bit by bit after some time, their staggering effect not seen until irreversible harm has been finished. While a youngster may rest every night with a full midsection, micronutrient lacks imply that their body is as yet hungry for good sustenance. A large number of youngsters experience the ill effects of hindered development, psychological postponements, debilitated insusceptibility and disease because of micronutrient insufficiencies. For pregnant ladies, the absence of basic nutrients and minerals can be calamitous, expanding the danger of low birth weight, birth deformities, stillbirth, and even passing.

Macronutrients versus micronutrients

Dissimilar to macronutrients, micronutrients (Vitamins and minerals) are required in exceptionally modest quantities however are as yet important for typical body working. They empower numerous concoction responses in the body however don't give calories. Vitamins are basic for typical digestion, development, and advancement, while minerals are predominantly required as co-factors or the capacity of proteins in the body. Concentrate on a wide assortment of vivid nourishments to meet your microVitamin standard. Macrominerals are required in bigger sums than trace minerals so as to play out their particular jobs in your body. The macrominerals and a portion of their capacities are the most needed nutrients for the body.

Mineral (supplement) and Composition of the human body

Dietary minerals are inorganic supplements and components required by living organisms, other than the four components carbon, hydrogen, nitrogen, and oxygen that are available in about every single natural particle. The expression "mineral" is antiquated, since the expectation is to portray essentially the less normal components in the eating regimen. Some are heavier than the four just referenced, including a few metals, which frequently happen as particles in the body. A few dietitians prescribe that these be provided from nourishments in which they happen normally, or if nothing else as intricate mixes, or once in a while even from common inorganic sources, (for example, calcium carbonate from ground clam shells). A few minerals are consumed considerably more promptly in the ionic structures found in such sources. Then again, minerals are regularly falsely added to the eating regimen as enhancements; the most renowned is likely iodine in iodized salt which avoids goiter.

Macrominerals

Numerous components are fundamental supplements called dietary minerals. Some have jobs as cofactors, while others are electrolytes.[74] Elements with prescribed dietary remittance (RDA) more prominent than 150 mg/day are, in order request:

Calcium, a typical electrolyte, yet in addition required fundamentally (for muscle and stomach related framework health, bone quality, a few structures kill causticity, gives flagging particles to nerve and layer capacities)

Chloride; major electrolyte

Magnesium, required for preparing ATP and related responses (constructs bone, encourages peristalsis)

Phosphorus, required segment of bones; fundamental

for vitality processing

Potassium, an electrolyte (heart and nerve capacities)

Sodium, an electrolyte; regular in nourishment and made drinks, normally as sodium chloride. Over the top sodium utilization can exhaust calcium and magnesium,[76] prompting hypertension.

Trace minerals

Numerous components are required in trace sums, as a rule since they assume a reactant job in enzymes. Some trace mineral components (RDA < 200 mg/day) are, in sequential order request:

Cobalt required for biosynthesis of Vitamin B12 group of coenzymes. Creatures can't biosynthesize B12, and must get this cobalt-containing Vitamin in their eating regimen.

Copper required part of numerous redox compounds, including cytochrome c oxidase.

Chromium required for sugar digestion

Iodine required for the biosynthesis of thyroxine as well as — it is assumed — for other significant organs as bosom, stomach, salivary organs, thymus, and so forth (see Extrathyroidal iodine); hence iodine is required in bigger amounts than others in this rundown, and in some cases characterized with the macrominerals.

Iron required for some compounds, and for hemoglobin and some different proteins

Manganese (preparing of oxygen)

Molybdenum required for xanthine oxidase and related oxidases

Selenium required for peroxidase (cancer prevention agent proteins)

Zinc required for a few catalysts, for example, carboxypeptidase, liver liquor dehydrogenase, and carbonic anhydrase

Vitamins

Vitamins are basic Vitamins, vital in the eating routine for good health. (Vitamin D is an exemption, as it very well may be incorporated in the skin within the sight of UVB radiation, and numerous creature species can integrate Vitamin C.) Vitamin lacks may bring about sickness conditions, including goiter, scurvy, osteoporosis, disabled safe framework, issue of cell digestion, certain types of malignancy, side effects of untimely maturing, and poor mental health, among numerous others. Excess degrees of certain Vitamins are additionally hazardous to health. The Food and Nutrition Board of the Institute of Medicine has set up Tolerable Upper Intake Levels (ULs) for seven vitamins. Micronutrients are dietary segments, frequently alluded to as Vitamins and minerals, which albeit just required by the body in limited quantities, are essential to advancement, ailment aversion, and prosperity. Micronutrients are not created in the body and should be gotten from the diet. Lacks in micronutrients, for example, iron, iodine, Vitamin A, folate and zinc can have destroying outcomes. At any rate half of kids overall ages a half year to 5 years experience the ill effects of at least one microVitamin insufficiency, and comprehensively in excess of 2 billion individuals are affected.

Vitamin A

Vitamin An is important to help sound visual perception and insusceptible framework capacities; youngsters who are lacking face an expanded danger of visual deficiency and demise from contaminations, for example, measles and diarrhea. Comprehensively, 1 of every 3 pre-school matured youngsters and 1 out of 6 pregnant ladies are Vitamin A lacking because of insufficient dietary intake. Vitamin A supplementation of kids 6-59 months has been demonstrated to be exceptionally compelling in lessening mortality from all causes in nations where Vitamin A lack is a general health concern.

Water-Soluble Vitamins

Most Vitamins break down in water and are in this manner known as water-solvent. They're not effectively put away in your body and get flushed out with urine when devoured in overabundance. While each water-solvent Vitamin has an exceptional job, their capacities are connected. For instance, most B Vitamins go about as coenzymes that help trigger significant synthetic responses. A great deal of these responses are fundamental for vitality creation.

The water-dissolvable Vitamins — with a portion of their capacities — are:

- Vitamin B1 (thiamine): Helps convert supplements into vitality

- Vitamin B2 (riboflavin): Necessary for vitality generation, cell capacity and fat digestion

- Vitamin B3 (niacin): Drives the creation of vitality from nourishment

- Vitamin B5 (pantothenic corrosive): Necessary for unsaturated fat combination

- Vitamin B6 (pyridoxine): Helps your body discharge sugar from put away starches for vitality and make red platelets

- Vitamin B7 (biotin): Plays a job in the digestion of unsaturated fats, amino acids and glucose

- Vitamin B9 (folate): Important for legitimate cell division

- Vitamin B12 (cobalamin): Necessary for red platelet development and appropriate sensory system and mind work

- Vitamin C (ascorbic corrosive): Required for the making of synapses and collagen, the principle protein in your skin

As should be obvious, water-dissolvable Vitamins assume a significant job in creating vitality yet in addition have a few different capacities. Since these Vitamins are not put away in your body, it's essential to get enough of them from nourishment.

Sources and Recommended Dietary

Allowances (RDAs) or Adequate Intakes (AIs) of water-dissolvable Vitamins are:

Vitamin	Sources	RDA or AI (grown-ups > 19 years)
Vitamin B1 (thiamine)	Whole grains, meat, fish	1.1–1.2 mg
Vitamin B2 (riboflavin)	Organ meats, eggs, milk	1.1–1.3 mg
Vitamin B3 (niacin)	Meat, salmon, verdant greens, beans	14–16 mg
Vitamin B5 (pantothenic acid)	Organ meats, mushrooms, fish, avocado	5 mg
Vitamin B6 (pyridoxine)	Fish, milk, carrots, potatoes	1.3 mg
Vitamin B7 (biotin)	Eggs, almonds, spinach, sweet potatoes	30 mg
Vitamin B9 (folate)	Beef, liver, dark looked at peas, spinach,	400 mg

	asparagus	
Vitamin B12 (cobalamin)	Clams, fish, meat	2.4 mg
Vitamin C (ascorbic acid)	Citrus natural products, chime peppers, Brussels sprouts	75–90 mg

Fat-Soluble Vitamins

Fat-solvent Vitamins don't break down in water. They're best ingested when expended close by a source of fat. After utilization, fat-solvent Vitamins are put away in your liver and fatty tissues for sometime later.

The names and elements of fat-solvent Vitamins are:

- Vitamin A: Necessary for legitimate vision and organ work

- Vitamin D: Promotes appropriate safe capacity and aids calcium retention and bone development.

- Vitamin E: Assists invulnerable capacity and goes about as a cancer prevention agent that shields cells from harm.

- Vitamin K: Required for blood thickening and legitimate bone advancement.

Sources and prescribed admissions of fat-solvent Vitamins are

Vitamin	Sources	RDA or AI (grown-ups > 19 years)
Vitamin A	Retinol (liver, dairy, fish), carotenoids (sweet potatoes, carrots, spinach)	700–900 mcg
Vitamin D	Sunlight, fish oil, milk	600–800 IU
Vitamin E	Sunflower seeds, wheat germ, almonds	15 mg
Vitamin K	Leafy greens, soybeans, pumpkin	90–120 mcg

Impact centers fundamentally around taking out inadequacies in iron, iodine, folate and zinc.

Iron

Iron is a basic mineral basic for engine and subjective advancement. Youngsters and pregnant ladies are particularly powerless against the outcomes of iron deficiency. Low hemoglobin fixation (iron deficiency) influences 43% of kids 5 years old and 38% of pregnant ladies globally. Iron deficiency during pregnancy builds the danger of maternal and perinatal mortality and low birth weight. Maternal and neonatal passings are a significant reason for mortality, together causing between 2.5 million and 3.4 million passings worldwide. WHO suggests iron and folic corrosive enhancements for lessening sickliness and improving iron status among ladies of conceptive age.

Flour fortress with iron and folic corrosive is internationally perceived as one of the best and minimal effort micronutrients interventions. Counteracting iron inadequacy improves youngsters' learning capacity and psychological advancement.

Iodine

Iodine is one of the most significant minerals required by a baby for mind and subjective improvement, however the iodine content in many nourishments and refreshments is low. 18 million infants are brought into the world rationally hindered on account of maternal iodine insufficiency and 38 million are conceived in danger of iodine deficiency9. All inclusive it is assessed that 2 billion individuals have deficient iodine intake. Stronghold of salt with iodine has been one of the best sustenance intercessions to date–71% of worldwide families approach iodized salt. Salt iodization has prompted an expansion in IQ focuses and critical decrease in the predominance of iodine lack issue, for example, goitres

Zinc

Zinc is a mineral that advances invulnerability, protection from contamination, and appropriate development and improvement of the anxious system, and is fundamental to solid pregnancy outcomes.17.3% of the worldwide populace is in danger for zinc insufficiency because of dietary deficiency, however up to 30% of individuals are in danger in certain districts of the world. Zinc supplementation lessens the rate of untimely birth, diminishes youth the runs and respiratory contaminations, brings down all-cause mortality, and builds development and weight gain among newborn children and youthful children

Folate

Folate is a Vitamin that is basic in the most punctual long periods of fetal development for solid improvement of the cerebrum, spinal string, and skull. Guaranteeing adequate degrees of folate in ladies preceding origination can lessen neural cylinder surrenders (a genuine birth imperfection) by up to 50%13. Supplementations of ladies 15-49 years with folic corrosive, and stronghold of nourishments, for example, wheat flour with folic corrosive, are viable intercessions for the decrease of birth imperfections, dreariness, and mortality in newborns.

Minerals are found in a scope of nourishment types. Dietary minerals are the other concoction components our bodies need, other than carbon, hydrogen, oxygen, and nitrogen. Individuals with a well-adjusted eating routine will, as a rule, acquire every one of the minerals they need from what they eat. Minerals are some of the time added to specific nourishments to compensate for any deficiencies. The best case of this is iodized salt - iodine is added to forestall iodine insufficiency, which influences around 2 billion people, all around; it causes mental impediment and thyroid organ issues. Iodine insufficiency stays a genuine general medical issue in over a large portion of the planet.

Specialists at the University of Florida state that key minerals are basic for human biochemical procedures:

Potassium

What it does - a foundational (influences whole body) electrolyte, basic in co-controlling ATP (a significant transporter of vitality in cells in the body, additionally key in making RNA) with sodium. Potassium: Electrolyte that keeps up liquid status in cells and assists with nerve transmission and muscle work.

Insufficiency - hypokalemia - can significantly influence the sensory system and heart.

Abundance - hyperkalemia - can likewise significantly influence the sensory system and heart.

Chloride

What it does - key for creating stomach corrosive, significant in the vehicle of atoms among cells, and imperative for the best possible working of nerves. Chloride is often found in blend with sodium. Keeps up liquid equalization and is utilized to make stomach related juices.

Lack - hypochloremia - low salt levels, which, if extreme, can be exceptionally risky.

Overabundance - hyperchloremia - for the most part no manifestations, connected with unreasonable liquid misfortune.

Sodium

What it does - a fundamental electrolyte, and basic in managing ATP with potassium. Significant for nerve capacity and controlling body liquid levels. Sodium is an electrolyte that guides liquid equalization and support of circulatory strain

Inadequacy - hyponatremia - makes cells glitch; incredibly low sodium can be deadly.

Overabundance - hypernatremia - can likewise make cells glitch, very significant levels can be deadly.

Calcium

What it does - significant for muscle, heart, and stomach related health. Manufactures bone, aids the amalgamation and capacity of platelets. It is necessary for appropriate structure and capacity of bones and teeth. Aids muscle capacity and vein withdrawall.

Inadequacy - hypocalcaemia - muscle cramps, stomach issues, fits, and hyperactive profound ligament reflexes.

Overabundance - hypercalcemia - muscle shortcoming, obstruction, undermined conduction of electrical driving forces in the heart, calcium stones in the urinary tract, debilitated kidney work, and hindered retention of iron, prompting iron lack.

Phosphorus

What it does - significant for the structure of DNA, transporter of vitality (ATP), segment of cell layer, fortifies bones.

Phosphorus: Part of bone and cell layer structure

Inadequacy - hypophosphatemia, a model is rickets.

Abundance - hyperphosphatemia, frequently a consequence of kidney disappointment.

Magnesium

What it does - forms ATP; required for good bones and the board of legitimate muscle development.

Many chemicals depend on magnesium to work appropriately.

Magnesium: Assists with more than 300 protein responses, including guideline of circulatory strain

Inadequacy - hypomagnesemia - urinevishness of the sensory system with fits of the hands and feet,

Sulfur: Part of each living tissue and contained in the amino acids methionine and cysteine

Sources and suggested admissions of the macrominerals are

Nutrients	Sources	RDA or AI (grown-ups > 19 years)
Calcium	Milk items, verdant greens, broccoli	2,000–2,500 mg
Phosphorus	Almonds, cashews, dark beans	700 mg
Magnesium	Salmon, yogurt, turkey	310–420 mg

Sodium	Salt, handled nourishments, canned soup	2,300 mg
Chloride	Seaweed, salt, celery	1,800–2,300 mg
Potassium	Lentils, oak seed squash, bananas	4,700 mg
Sulfur	Garlic, onions, Brussels grows, eggs, mineral water	None built up

Trace Minerals

Trace minerals are required in littler sums than macrominerals yet at the same time empower significant capacities in your body.

The trace minerals and a portion of their capacities are:

- Iron: Helps give oxygen to muscles and aids the production of specific hormones

- Manganese: Assists in starch, amino corrosive and cholesterol digestion

- Copper: Required for connective tissue

development, just as should be expected cerebrum and sensory system work

- Zinc: Necessary for ordinary development, resistant capacity and wound recuperating

- Iodine: Assists in thyroid guideline

- Fluoride: Necessary for the advancement of bones and teeth

- Selenium: Important for thyroid health, propagation and protection against oxidative harm

Sources and suggested admissions of trace minerals are

Nutrients	Sources	RDA or AI (grown-ups > 19 years)
Iron	Oysters, a health doctor beans, spinach	8–18 mg
Manganese	Pineapple, walnuts, peanuts	1.8–2.3 mg
Copper	Liver, crabs,	900 mcg

	cashews	
Zinc	Oysters, crab, chickpeas	8–11 mg
Iodine	Seaweed, cod, yogurt	150 mcg
Fluoride	Fruit juice, water, crab	3–4 mg
Selenium	Brazil nuts, sardines, ham	55 mcg

Synopsis – Micronutrients can be partitioned into four gatherings — water-solvent Vitamins, fat-dissolvable Vitamins, macrominerals and trace minerals. The capacities, nourishment sources and prescribed admissions of every Vitamin and mineral fluctuate.

Medical advantages of micronutrient

All micronutrient are critical for the correct working of your body.

Devouring a sufficient measure of the various Vitamins and minerals is vital to ideal health and may even help battle ailment.

This is on the grounds that micronutrient are a piece of almost every procedure in your body. In addition, certain Vitamins and minerals can go about as cancer prevention agents.

Cancer prevention agents may ensure against cell harm that has been related with specific maladies, including malignancy, Alzheimer's and coronary illness.

For instance, inquire about has connected a sufficient dietary admission of Vitamins An and C with a lower danger of certain kinds of malignancy.

Getting enough of certain Vitamins may likewise help counteract Alzheimer's ailment. An audit of seven examinations found that sufficient dietary admission of Vitamins E, C and An is related with a 24%, 17% and 12% decreased danger of creating Alzheimer's, individually.

CHAPTER TEN

NUTRITION DISORDERS

As per WHO, lack of healthy sustenance alludes to inadequacies, abundances, or awkward nature in an individual's admission of vitality and additionally supplements. The term hunger tends to 3 general gatherings of conditions: undernutrition, which incorporates squandering (low weight-for-tallness), hindering (low stature for-age) and underweight (low weight-for-age); microVitamin-related ailing health, which incorporates microVitamin inadequacies or insuficiencies (an absence of significant Vitamins and minerals) or microVitamin abundance; and overweight, obesity and diet-related noncommunicable illnesses, (for example, coronary illness, stroke, diabetes and some cancers). In Mali, the International Crops Research Institute for the Semi-Arid Tropics (ICRISAT) and the Aga Khan Foundation prepared ladies' gatherings to make equinut, a solid and nourishing variant of the conventional formula di-dèguè (containing nut glue, nectar and millet or rice flour). The point was to support sustenance and vocations by creating an item that ladies could make and sell, and which would be acknowledged by the neighborhood network in light of its nearby heritage.

Insufficient

The U.S. Nourishment and Nutrition Board sets Estimated Average Requirements (EARs) and Recommended Dietary Allowances (RDAs) for Vitamins and minerals. EARs and RDAs are a piece of Dietary Reference Intakes. The DRI records depict supplement lack signs and indications.

Excessive

The U.S. Nourishment and Nutrition Board sets Tolerable Upper Intake Levels (known as ULs) for Vitamins and minerals when proof is adequate. ULs are set a protected division underneath sums appeared to mess health up. ULs are a piece of Dietary Reference Intakes. The European Food Safety Authority additionally surveys a similar security questions and set its own ULs.

Unbalanced

At the point when a lot of at least one supplements is available in the eating routine to the prohibition of the correct measure of different supplements, the eating routine is said to be unequal. Fatty nourishment fixings, for example, vegetable oils, sugar and liquor are alluded to as "unfilled calories" since they dislodge from the eating regimen food sources that likewise contain protein, Vitamins, minerals and fiber.

Health Deficiencies

Regardless of whether you are getting enough to eat, on the off chance that you are not eating a reasonable eating regimen, you may in any case be in danger for certain dietary inadequacies. Likewise, you may have dietary inadequacies because of certain health or life conditions, for example, pregnancy, or certain meds you might be taking, for example, hypertension drugs. Individuals who have had intestinal ailments or had areas of digestion tracts evacuated because of infection or weight reduction medical procedure likewise might be in danger for Vitamin insufficiencies. Heavy drinkers are likewise at high danger of having dietary insufficiencies.

One of the most well-known healthful inadequacies is iron insufficiency paleness. Your platelets need iron so as to supply your body with oxygen, and in the event that you need more iron, your blood won't work appropriately. Other dietary insufficiencies that can influence your platelets incorporate low degrees of Vitamin B12, folate, or Vitamin C.

Vitamin D inadequacy may influence the soundness of your bones, making it hard for you to assimilate and utilize calcium (another mineral that you may not be getting enough of). In spite of the fact that you can get Vitamin D by going out in the sun, numerous individuals with worries about skin malignant growth may wind up with low degrees of Vitamin D by not getting enough sun.

Other healthful lacks include:

Beriberi	Low degrees of Vitamin B1 (found in grain husks)
Ariboflavin osis	Low degrees of Vitamin B2
Pellagra	Low degrees of Vitamin B3
Paraesthesi a	Low degrees of Vitamin B5 prompting a "tingling sensation" feeling
Biotin lack	Low degrees of Vitamin B7, which can be normal in pregnancy
Hypocobal aminemia	Low degrees of B12

Night visual deficiency	Low degrees of Vitamin A
Scurvy	Low degrees of Vitamin C
Rickets	Extreme Vitamin D and additionally calcium lack

Vitamin K inadequacy : happens with specific prescriptions and restorative issues

magnesium inadequacy: happens with specific prescriptions and restorative issues

potassium inadequacy: happens with specific prescriptions and restorative issues

Eating a reasonable eating routine can help anticipate these conditions. Vitamin enhancements might be fundamental for specific individuals, for example, pregnant or nursing moms and individuals with intestinal conditions.

Ailments and Conditions Influenced by Nutrition

Numerous health conditions are caused and additionally influenced by nourishment and sustenance. Some are legitimately brought about by nourishment, for example, "food contamination" or bacterial diseases from polluted nourishment. A few people can have extreme hypersensitivities to nourishments like peanuts, shellfish, or wheat (celiac infection). Gastrointestinal sicknesses, for example, bad tempered entrail disorder, ulcerative colitis, and gastroesophageal reflux infection (GERD)— are additionally straightforwardly influenced by the utilization of nourishment. For different infections and conditions, the sort or amount of nourishment can impact the advancement of the ailment. Diabetes mellitus, for instance, which brings about the failure of the body to control glucose, is radically influenced by the sorts and amounts of nourishment eaten. Starch admission must be painstakingly observed on the off chance that you experience the ill effects of diabetes, or glucose can ascend to perilous levels. Different conditions influenced by nourishment and sustenance include:

- Hypertension: Salt admission influences circulatory strain.

- Coronary illness/elevated cholesterol: Fatty nourishments and fractional hydrogenated oils can make plaque in supply routes.

- Osteoporosis: Low calcium, low Vitamin D and overabundance fat can bring about delicate bones.

- Certain malignant growths: A terrible eating routine and weight are related with expanded danger of bosom, colon, endometrial, esophageal, and kidney tumors.

Your nourishment decisions and dietary status can impact your general health over the whole course of your life.

Different Considerations

For specific sicknesses, deciding to eat certain nourishments and take certain enhancements may assist you with keeping up your health. Patients experiencing malignant growth treatment may require a particular eating routine so as to keep up their stamina. For example, unhealthy nourishments may should be expended to look after vitality. Getting enough calories and protein in the eating routine can conceivably help with long haul endurance.

Regardless, what you eat can help lessen your medical issues. Studies have indicated that on the off chance that you experience the ill effects of gout, eating fruits routinely can lessen your odds of a gout assault (Zhang, 2012). Garlic might be a full of feeling drug against specific microscopic organisms and parasites (Ankri et al., 1999). Nectar has antimicrobial and mitigating properties (Bogdanov et al., 2008). Expending apples may really lessen your hazard for colorectal malignant growth (Jedrychowski et al., 2009Trusted Source). Furthermore, drinking enough water rather than sweet pop or squeeze can help with weight control, appearance, and generally speaking protection from illness (Popkin et al., 2010).

Hoping to curtail sugar? We'll give you some sweet tips. Our Nutrition bulletin's multi day sugar challenge guides you in acquiring more attention to the sugars the nourishments you eat and gives you the devices you have to settle on more beneficial options. We should begin!

Vegetable and seed oils are profoundly handled oils that are effectively harmed during cooking. A few investigations propose that they can cause hurt and contribute. Purple cabbage is an adaptable vegetable that preferences like green cabbage however is more extravagant in useful plant mixes. Here are 8 amazing...

Sticks and jams are both adored, sweet spreads, however you may think about what separates them. This article audits the similitudes and contrasts...

Not all high protein nourishments are made equivalent. The 10 nourishments on this rundown are amazingly high in this supplement, involving only protein and...

The nourishments that a dairy animals eats can fundamentally influence its meat's supplement organization. This article clarifies the contrast among grass-and grain-bolstered

Orthorexia nervosa is a dietary problem that includes a fixation on good dieting.

Garlic is a heavenly and regular fixing that adds flavor and profundity to numerous dishes. This article surveys the most ideal approaches to store garlic.

Nourishment Deficiencies

Nourishment deficiencies, any of the supplement related infections and conditions that reason disease in people. They may remember lacks or overabundances for the eating routine, heftiness and dietary problems, and constant sicknesses, for example, cardiovascular ailment, hypertension, malignancy, and diabetes mellitus. Wholesome ailments additionally incorporate formative irregularities that can be anticipated by diet, genetic metabolic issue that react to dietary treatment, the communication of nourishments and supplements with drugs, nourishment hypersensitivities and bigotries, and potential risks in the nourishment supply. These classifications are depicted in this article. For a discourse of fundamental supplements, dietary suggestions, and human healthful needs and worries for the duration of the existence cycle, see nourishment, human.

Supplement Deficiencies

In spite of the fact that the alleged sicknesses of human progress—for instance, coronary illness, stroke, malignant growth, and diabetes—will be the focal point of this article, the most huge nourishment related ailment is interminable undernutrition, which torment in excess of 925 million individuals around the world. Undernutrition is a condition wherein there is inadequate nourishment to address vitality issues; its principle attributes incorporate weight reduction, inability to flourish, and squandering of muscle versus fat and muscle. Low birth weight in newborn children, insufficient development and improvement in kids, lessened mental capacity, and expanded defenselessness to illness are among the numerous results of constant diligent craving, which influences those living in destitution in both industrialized and creating nations. The biggest number of incessantly hungry individuals live in Asia, yet the seriousness of yearning is most prominent in sub-Saharan Africa. Toward the beginning of the 21st century, roughly 20,000 individuals, most of them kids, kicked the bucket every day from undernutrition and related sicknesses that could have been anticipated. The passings of a significant number of these youngsters originate from the poor nourishing status of their moms, just as the absence of chance forced by neediness.

Just a little level of yearning passings is brought about by starvation because of cataclysmic nourishment deficiencies. During the 1990s, for instance, overall starvation (scourge disappointment of the nourishment supply) all the more frequently came about because of complex social and political issues and the assaults of war than from catastrophic events, for example, dry seasons and floods.

Lack of healthy sustenance is the debilitated capacity

that outcomes from a drawn out inadequacy—or overabundance—of all out vitality or explicit supplements, for example, protein, basic unsaturated fats, Vitamins, or minerals. This condition can come about because of fasting and anorexia nervosa; determined heaving (as in bulimia nervosa) or failure to swallow; weakened processing and intestinal malabsorption; or incessant sicknesses that outcome in loss of craving (e.g., malignant growth, AIDS). Lack of healthy sustenance can likewise result from restricted nourishment accessibility, impulsive nourishment decisions, or enthusiastic utilization of dietary enhancements.

Chosen lack of nutrient caused sicknesses are recorded in the table

sickness (and key supplement involved)	symptoms
xerophthalmia (Vitamin A)	blindness from interminable eye diseases, poor development, dryness and keratinization of epithelial tissues

	liver
rickets (Vitamin D)	weakened bones, bowed legs, other bone deformities
beriberi (thiamin)	nerve degeneration, modified muscle coordination, cardiovascular problems
pellagra (niacin)	diarrhea, skin irritation, dementia mushrooms
scurvy (Vitamin C)	delayed wound recuperating, inward dying, irregular arrangement of bones and teeth
iron-insufficiency frailty (iron)	decreased work yield, decreased development, expanded health hazard in pregnancy
goiter (iodine)	enlarged thyroid organ, poor development in outset

	and youth, conceivable mental impediment, cretinism

Protein-vitality ailing health

Constant undernutrition shows principally as protein-vitality lack of healthy sustenance (PEM), which is the most widely recognized type of ailing health around the world. Otherwise called protein-calorie ailing health, PEM is a continuum where individuals—very frequently youngsters—expend too little protein, vitality, or both. Toward one side of the continuum is kwashiorkor, described by a serious protein insufficiency, and at the other is marasmus, an outright nourishment hardship with terribly deficient measures of both vitality and protein.

A baby with marasmus is very underweight and has lost most or all subcutaneous fat. The body has a "skin and bones" appearance, and the youngster is significantly powerless and exceptionally defenseless to diseases. The reason is an eating routine exceptionally low in calories from all sources (counting protein), regularly from early weaning to a packaged recipe arranged with perilous water and weakened in view of destitution. Poor cleanliness and proceeded with exhaustion lead to an endless loop of gastroenteritis and decay of the coating of the gastrointestinal tract, which meddles with assimilation of supplements from the little nourishment accessible and further diminishes protection from disease. On the off chance that untreated, marasmus may bring about death because of starvation or cardiovascular breakdown.

Kwashiorkor, a Ghanaian word meaning the illness that the main kid gets when the new youngster comes, is regularly observed when a kid is weaned from high-protein bosom milk onto a starch nourishment source with inadequate protein. Youngsters with this illness, which is portrayed by a swollen tummy because of edema (liquid maintenance), are feeble, develop ineffectively, and are progressively defenseless to irresistible sicknesses, which may bring about deadly looseness of the bowels. Different side effects of kwashiorkor incorporate unresponsiveness, hair staining, and dry, stripping skin with wounds that neglect to recuperate. Weight reduction might be camouflaged due to the nearness of edema, expanded fatty liver, and intestinal parasites; additionally, there might be small squandering of muscle and muscle to fat ratio.

Kwashiorkor and marasmus can likewise happen in hospitalized patients accepting intravenous glucose for an all-encompassing time, as while recouping from medical procedure, or in those with ailments causing loss of hunger or malabsorption of supplements. People with dietary issues, malignant growth, AIDS, and different ailments where hunger falls flat or ingestion of supplements is hampered may lose muscle and organ tissue just as fat stores.

Treatment of PEM has three segments. Life-undermining conditions, for example, liquid and electrolyte irregular characteristics and contaminations—must be settled. Nutritional status ought to be reestablished as fast and securely as could be expected under the circumstances; quick weight addition can happen in a destitute kid inside half a month. he focal point of treatment at that point movements to guaranteeing dietary restoration as long as possible. The surined and extreme achievement of recuperation rely on the seriousness of lack of healthy sustenance, the practicality of treatment, and the ampleness of continuous help. Especially during the primary year of life, starvation may bring about decreased mind development and scholarly working that can't be completely reestablished.

Carbohydrates

Under most conditions, there is no outright dietary prerequisite for sugars—straightforward sugars, complex starches, for example, starches, and the toxic plant sugars known as dietary fiber. Certain cells, for example, synapses, require the basic sugar glucose as fuel. On the off chance that dietary starch is lacking, glucose amalgamation relies upon the breakdown of amino acids got from body protein and dietary protein and the compound glycerol, which is gotten from fat. Long haul sugar deficiency brings about expanded creation of natural mixes called ketones (a condition known as ketosis), which confers a particular sweet scent to the breath. Ketosis and other untoward impacts of an extremely low-starch diet can be avoided by the day by day utilization of 50 to 100 grams of sugar; be that as it may, getting in any event half of the every day vitality admission from sugars is suggested and is commonplace of human weight control plans, comparing to at any rate 250 grams of starch (1,000 calories in a 2,000-calorie diet). A fluctuated eating routine containing natural products, vegetables, vegetables, and entire grain oats, which are on the whole bottomless in starches, likewise gives an attractive admission of dietary fiber.

Basic unsaturated fats

There is likewise a base prerequisite for fat—not for all out fat, yet just for the unsaturated fats linoleic corrosive (a purported omega-6 unsaturated fat) and alpha-linolenic corrosive (an omega-3 unsaturated fat). Insufficiencies of these two unsaturated fats have been seen in hospitalized patients nourished only with intravenous liquids containing no fat for a considerable length of time, patients with ailments influencing fat retention, newborn children given recipes low in fat, and small kids bolstered nonfat milk or low-fat eating regimens. Side effects of lack incorporate dry skin, male pattern baldness, and disabled injury mending. Fundamental unsaturated fat necessities—a couple of grams daily—can be met by expending roughly a tablespoon of polyunsaturated plant oils day by day. fatty fish likewise gives a rich source of omega-3 unsaturated fats. Indeed, even people traceing a low-fat eating routine for the most part devour adequate fat to meet prerequisites.

Vitamins

In spite of the fact that insufficiency illnesses have been depicted in lab creatures and people denied of single Vitamins, in human experience various lacks are generally present all the while. The eight B-complex Vitamins work in coordination in various compound frameworks and metabolic pathways; in this way, an inadequacy of one may influence the working of others.

- Vitamin A

Vitamin An inadequacy is the main source of preventable visual impairment in kids and is a significant issue in the creating scene, particularly in Africa and Southeast Asia; in the most unfortunate nations a huge number of kids become daze every year because of a lack of the Vitamin. Indeed, even a mellow inadequacy can debilitate insusceptible capacity, accordingly decreasing protection from illness. Night visual impairment is an early indication of Vitamin An inadequacy, trailed by unusual dryness of the eye and at last scarring of the cornea, a condition known as xerophthalmia. Different indications incorporate dry skin, solidifying of epithelial cells somewhere else in the body, (for example, mucous films), and hindered development and improvement. In numerous regions where Vitamin A lack is endemic, the rate is being diminished by giving kids a solitary enormous portion of Vitamin An at regular intervals. A hereditarily adjusted type of rice containing beta-carotene, a forerunner of Vitamin A, can possibly lessen extraordinarily the rate of Vitamin An insufficiency, however the utilization of this purported brilliant rice is dubious.

* Vitamin D

Vitamin D (otherwise called Vitamin D hormone) is orchestrated in the body in a progression of steps, beginning in the skin by the activity of daylight's bright beams on an antecedent compound; in this manner, without sufficient nourishment sources of Vitamin D, an inadequacy of the Vitamin can happen when presentation to daylight is constrained. Absence of Vitamin D in kids causes rickets, an ailment portrayed by deficient mineralization of bone, development impediment, and skeletal disfigurements, for example, bowed legs. The grown-up type of rickets, known as osteomalacia, brings about powerless muscles just as feeble bones. Lacking Vitamin D may likewise add to the diminishing of bones found in osteoporosis. People with restricted sun introduction (counting ladies who totally spread their bodies for strict reasons), old or homebound people, and those with dull skin, especially the individuals who live in northern scopes, are in danger of Vitamin D inadequacy. Vitamin D is found in not many nourishments normally; therefore fortress of milk and different nourishments (e.g., margarine, oats, and breads) with the Vitamin has ensured those populaces where sun presentation is insufficient. Supplemental Vitamin D likewise may help secure against bone cracks in the old, who make and actuate Vitamin D less proficiently regardless of whether presented to daylight.

- Vitamin E

Vitamin E lack is uncommon in people, despite the fact that it might create in untimely newborn children and in individuals with debilitated fat assimilation or digestion. In the previous, delicacy of red platelets (hemolysis) is seen; in the last mentioned, where insufficiency is increasingly drawn out, neuromuscular brokenness including the spinal line and retina may bring about loss of reflexes, disabled parity and coordination, muscle shortcoming, and visual unsettling influences. No particular metabolic capacity has been set up for Vitamin E; be that as it may, it is a significant piece of the cancer prevention agent framework that restrains lipid peroxidation; i.e., it secures cells and their films against the harming impacts of free radicals (receptive oxygen and nitrogen species) that are delivered metabolically or enter the body from the earth. The prerequisite for Vitamin E is expanded with expanding utilization of polyunsaturated unsaturated fats. Individuals who smoke or are exposed to air contamination may likewise require a greater amount of the Vitamin to secure against oxidative harm to the lungs.

- Vitamin K

Vitamin K is essential for the development of prothrombin and other blood-coagulating factors in the liver, and it likewise assumes a job in bone digestion. A type of the Vitamin is delivered by microscopic organisms in the colon and can be used somewhat. Vitamin K inadequacy causes disabled coagulating of the blood and inward dying, even without damage. Because of poor vehicle of Vitamin K over the placenta, babies in created nations are routinely given the Vitamin intramuscularly or orally inside six hours of birth to ensure against a condition known as hemorrhagic infection of the infant. Vitamin K lack is uncommon in grown-ups, aside from in disorders with poor fat retention, in liver ailment, or during treatment with certain anticoagulant drugs, which meddle with Vitamin K digestion. Seeping because of Vitamin K insufficiency might be found in patients whose gut microscopic organisms have been slaughtered by anti-microbials.

- Thiamin

Drawn out insufficiency of thiamin (Vitamin B1) brings about beriberi, a sickness that has been endemic in populaces where a health doctor rice has been the staple. Thiamin lack is still found in territories where a health doctor rice or flour establishes the greater part of the eating routine and thiamin lost in processing isn't supplanted through improvement. Indications of the structure known as dry beriberi incorporate loss of craving, disarray and other mental manifestations, muscle shortcoming, agonizing lower leg muscles, poor coordination, shivering and loss of motion. In wet beriberi there is edema and the plausibility of an extended heart and cardiovascular breakdown. Thiamin inadequacy can likewise happen in populaces eating huge amounts of crude fish harboring intestinal organisms that contain the catalyst thiaminase. In the created world, thiamin inadequacy is connected fundamentally to ceaseless liquor abuse with less than stellar eating routine, showing as Wernicke-Korsakoff disorder, a condition with quick eye developments, loss of muscle coordination, mental perplexity, and memory misfortune.

- Riboflavin

Riboflavin (Vitamin B2) lack, known as ariboflavinosis, is improbable without the synchronous insufficiency of different supplements. traceing a while of riboflavin hardship, indications remember breaks for the skin at the edges of the mouth, gaps of the lips, and a kindled, fuchsia hued tongue. Since riboflavin is promptly decimated by bright light, embittered newborn children who are treated with light treatment are directed the Vitamin. Milk, milk items, and grains, significant sources of riboflavin in the eating regimen, are bundled to avoid introduction to light.

- Vitamin B12

Inadequacy of Vitamin B12 (cobalamin), like folic corrosive, brings about megaloblastic weakness (enormous, youthful red platelets), because of obstruction with typical DNA blend. Also, Vitamin B12 keeps up the myelin sheath that secures nerve strands; in this manner, an untreated insufficiency of the Vitamin can bring about nerve degeneration and inevitably loss of motion. A lot of folic corrosive (more than 1,000 µg every day) may cover, and perhaps even worsen, a basic Vitamin B12 lack. Just creature nourishments are dependable sources of Vitamin B12. Veggie lovers, who eat no nourishments of creature inception, are in danger of Vitamin B12 insufficiency and must get the Vitamin through invigorated nourishment or an enhancement. For individuals who normally eat creature items, inadequacy of the Vitamin is impossible, except if there is a deformity in retention. So as to be ingested, Vitamin B12 must be bound to natural factor, a substance emitted by the stomach. On the off chance that inborn factor is missing (because of an immune system issue known as poisonous sickliness) or if there is deficient creation of hydrochloric corrosive by the stomach, ingestion of the Vitamin will be constrained. Malicious paleness, which happens frequently in the old, can be treated by infusions or enormous oral portions (1,000 µg) of Vitamin B12.

- Pantothenic corrosive

Pantothenic corrosive is so across the board in nourishments that lack is far-fetched under typical conditions. Insufficiency has been seen distinctly in people nourished semisynthetic eating regimens inadequate in the Vitamin or in subjects given a pantothenic corrosive foe. Side effects of inadequacy incorporate weariness, crabbiness, rest unsettling influences, stomach trouble, and neurological side effects, for example, shivering in the hands. Lack of the Vitamin was suspected during World War II when detainees of war in Asia who displayed "consuming feet" disorder, described by deadness and shivering in the toes and other neurological indications, reacted uniquely to the organization of pantothenic corrosive.

- Biotin

Lack of biotin is uncommon, and this might be expected partially to union of the Vitamin by microscopic organisms in the colon, in spite of the fact that the significance of this source is hazy. Biotin inadequacy has been seen in individuals who routinely eat huge amounts of crude egg a health doctor, which contains a glycoprotein (avidin) that ties biotin and avoids its assimilation. An uncommon hereditary imperfection that renders a few newborn children incapable to retain a type of biotin in nourishment can be treated with an enhancement of the Vitamin. Long haul utilization of certain anticonvulsant medications may likewise disable biotin retention. Side effects of insufficiency incorporate skin rash, male pattern baldness, and in the end neurological variations from the norm.

- Vitamin C

Vitamin C, otherwise called ascorbic corrosive, works as a water-solvent cell reinforcement and as a cofactor in different catalyst frameworks, for example, those associated with the union of connective tissue parts and synapses. Manifestations of scurvy, a disease brought about by Vitamin C lack, incorporate pinpoint hemorrhages (petechiae) under the skin, draining gums, joint agony, and disabled injury recuperating. Albeit uncommon in created nations, scurvy is seen sporadically in individuals devouring confined weight control plans, especially those containing scarcely any foods grown from the ground, or in newborn children sustained heated up bovine's milk and no source of Vitamin C. Scurvy can be averted with moderately little amounts of Vitamin C (10 milligrams [mg] every day), in spite of the fact that prescribed admissions, which mean to give adequate cell reinforcement assurance, are more like 100 mg for each day. Infection states, ecological poisons, drugs, and different burdens can expand a person's Vitamin C needs. Smokers, for instance, may require an extra 35 mg of the Vitamin day by day to keep up Vitamin C levels practically identical to nonsmokers.

Minerals

Iron

Iron inadequacy is the most widely recognized of every wholesome lack, with a significant part of the total populace being inadequate in the mineral somewhat. Little youngsters and premenopausal ladies are the most powerless. The primary capacity of iron is in the arrangement of hemoglobin, the red color of the blood that conveys oxygen from the lungs to different tissues. Since every milliliter of blood contains 0.5 mg of iron (as a segment of hemoglobin), draining can deplete the body's iron stores. At the point when iron stores are exhausted a condition emerges known as microcytic hypochromic frailty, described by little red platelets that contain less hemoglobin than typical. Indications of serious iron lack sickliness incorporate weariness, shortcoming, disregard, fair skin, trouble breathing on effort, and low protection from cold temperatures. During youth, iron insufficiency can influence conduct and learning capacity just as development and improvement. Serious frailty builds the danger of pregnancy intricacies and maternal demise. Iron insufficiency sickliness is generally regular during late outset and early youth, when iron stores present from birth are depleted and milk, which is poor in iron, is an essential nourishment; during the pre-adult development spurt; and in ladies during the childbearing years, as a result of blood misfortune during period and the extra iron needs of pregnancy. Intestinal blood misfortune and ensuing iron insufficiency weakness in grown-ups may likewise originate from ulcers, hemorrhoids, tumors, or interminable utilization of specific medications, for example, ibuprofen. In creating nations, blood misfortune because of hookworm and different contaminations, combined with insufficient dietary iron admission, compounds iron lack in the two youngsters and grown-ups.

Iodine

Iodine insufficiency issue are the most widely recognized reason for preventable cerebrum harm, which influences an expected 50 million individuals around the world. During pregnancy, extreme iodine lack may weaken fetal improvement, bringing about cretinism (irreversible mental impediment with short stature and formative variations from the norm) just as in unnatural birth cycle and stillbirth. Other increasingly inescapable results of incessant iodine inadequacy incorporate lesser psychological and neuromuscular shortfalls. The sea is a reliable source of iodine, yet away from seaside territories iodine in nourishment is variable and generally mirrors the sum in the dirt. In interminable iodine inadequacy the thyroid organ expands as it endeavors to trap more iodide (the structure where iodine works in the body) from the blood for combination of thyroid hormones, and it in the end turns into an unmistakable knot at the front of the neck known as a goiter. A few nourishments, for example, cassava, millet, sweet potato, certain beans, and individuals from the cabbage family, contain substances known as goitrogens that meddle with thyroid hormone amalgamation; these substances, which are crushed by cooking, can be a huge factor in people with existing together iodine inadequacy who depend on goitrogenic food sources as staples. Since a methodology of widespread iodization of salt was embraced in 1993, there has been surprising advancement in improving iodine status around the world. In any case, a large number of individuals living in iodine-inadequate zones, essentially in

Central Africa, Southeast and Central Asia, and even in focal and eastern Europe, stay in danger.

Zinc

A constituent of various compounds, zinc assumes an auxiliary job in proteins and directs quality articulation. Zinc insufficiency in people was first revealed during the 1960s in Egypt and Iran, where youngsters and pre-adult young men with hindered development and lacking genitalia reacted to treatment with zinc. Insufficiency of the mineral was ascribed to the provincial eating routine, which was low in meat and high in vegetables, unleavened breads, and entire grain nourishments that contain fiber, phytic corrosive, and different variables that repress zinc ingestion. Likewise adding to zinc lack was the act of mud eating, which meddles with the assimilation of zinc, iron, and different minerals. Serious zinc lack has likewise been depicted in patients nourished intravenous arrangements insufficient in zinc and in the acquired zinc-responsive disorder known as acrodermatitis enteropathica. Indications of zinc inadequacy may incorporate skin injuries, looseness of the bowels, expanded defenselessness to contaminations, night visual impairment, diminished taste and smell sharpness, poor craving, balding, slow twisted mending, low sperm tally, and weakness. Zinc is most noteworthy in protein-rich nourishments, particularly red meat and shellfish, and zinc status might be low in protein-vitality hunger. Indeed, even in created nations, little youngsters, pregnant ladies, the older, exacting veggie lovers, individuals with liquor addiction, and those with malabsorption disorders are helpless against zinc lack

Fluoride

Fluoride additionally adds to the mineralization of bones and teeth and ensures against tooth rot. Epidemiological investigations in the United States during the 1930s and 1940s uncovered a backwards connection between the common fluoride substance of waters and the pace of dental caries. In zones where fluoride levels in the drinking water are low, remedy fluoride supplements are suggested for kids more established than a half year of age; dental specialists likewise may apply fluoride washes or gels occasionally to their patients' teeth. Fluoridated toothpastes are a significant source of fluoride for youngsters and furthermore for grown-ups, who keep on profiting by fluoride consumption.

Calcium

Practically all the calcium in the body is during the bones and teeth, the skeleton filling in as a repository for calcium required in the blood and somewhere else. During youth and youthfulness, sufficient calcium admission is basic for bone development and calcification. A low calcium consumption during adolescence, and particularly during the youthful development spurt, may incline one to osteoporosis, an illness described by decreased bone mass, further down the road. As bones lose thickness, they become delicate and unfit to withstand common strains; the subsequent breaks, especially of the hip, may cause debilitation and even passing. Osteoporosis is especially basic in postmenopausal ladies in modern social orders. Not a calcium-inadequacy illness as such, osteoporosis is firmly impacted by heredity; danger of the sickness can be reduced by guaranteeing satisfactory calcium consumption all through life and taking part in normal weight-bearing activity. Adequate calcium consumption in the prompt postmenopausal years appears to slow bone misfortune, despite the fact that not to a similar degree as do bone-monitoring drugs.

Sodium

Sodium is generally given in sufficient sums by

nourishment, even without included table salt (sodium chloride). Moreover, the body's sodium-protection components are exceptionally created, and consequently sodium inadequacy is uncommon, in any event, for those on low-sodium abstains from food. Sodium exhaustion may happen during delayed overwhelming perspiring, spewing, or loose bowels or on account of kidney ailment. Indications of hyponatremia, or low blood sodium, incorporate muscle cramps, queasiness, wooziness, shortcoming, and in the end stun and extreme lethargies. After delayed high-power effort in the warmth, sodium equalization can be reestablished by drinking refreshments containing sodium and glucose (alleged games drinks) and by eating salted nourishment. Drinking a liter of water containing two milliliters (33% teaspoon) of table salt additionally should get the job done.

Chlorine

Chloride is lost from the body under conditions that parallel those of sodium misfortune. Serious chloride exhaustion brings about a condition known as metabolic alkalosis (overabundance alkalinity in body liquids).

Potassium

Potassium is generally dispersed in nourishments and is once in a while lacking in the eating regimen. In any case, a few diuretics utilized in the treatment of hypertension drain potassium. The mineral is additionally lost during supported heaving or the runs or with constant utilization of diuretics. Indications of potassium insufficiency incorporate shortcoming, loss of hunger, muscle issues, and perplexity. Extreme hypokalemia (low blood potassium) may bring about heart arrhythmias. Potassium-rich nourishments, for example, bananas or oranges, can help supplant misfortunes of the mineral, as can potassium chloride supplements, which ought to be taken distinctly under therapeutic supervision.

Water inadequacy (lack of hydration)

Water is the biggest segment of the body, representing the greater part of body weight. To supplant liquid misfortunes, grown-ups by and large need to devour 2 to 4 liters of liquid day by day in cool atmospheres, contingent upon level of movement, and from 8 to 16 liters every day in extremely hot atmospheres. Drying out may create if water utilization neglects to fulfill thirst; if the thirst system isn't working appropriately, as during

168

extraordinary physical exercise; or if there is extreme liquid misfortune, similarly as with the runs or retching. When thirst is clear, there is some level of lack of hydration, which is characterized as loss of liquid adding up to in any event 1 to 2 percent of body weight. Side effects can advance rapidly if not revised: dry mouth, indented eyes, poor skin turgor, cold hands and feet, feeble and fast heartbeat, quick and shallow breathing, perplexity, weariness, and trance like state. Loss of liquid establishing in excess of 10 percent of body weight might be deadly. The old (whose thirst sensation might be dulled), individuals who are sick, and those flying in planes are particularly defenseless against drying out. Newborn children and youngsters with ceaseless undernutrition who create gastroenteritis may turn out to be seriously got dried out from loose bowels or regurgitating. Treatment is with an intravenous or oral arrangement of glucose and salts.

Supplement Toxicities

The requirement for every supplement falls inside a sheltered or attractive range, above which there is a danger of unfriendly impacts. Any supplement, even water, can be harmful whenever taken in extremely huge amounts. Overdoses of specific supplements, for example, iron, can cause harming (intense poisonous quality) and even passing. For most supplements, ongoing abundance consumption represents a danger of unfriendly health impacts (ceaseless lethality). Supported overconsumption of the calorie-yielding supplements (sugar, fat, and protein) and liquor builds the danger of weight and explicit interminable ailments (see beneath), and utilization of detached amino acids can prompt uneven characters and toxicities. Be that as it may, for most people, the danger of damage because of overabundance admission of Vitamins or minerals in nourishment is low. In 1997 the U.S. Organization of Medicine built up a reference esteem called the Tolerable Upper Intake Level (UL) for chose supplements, which is likewise being utilized as a model for different nations. The UL is the most significant level of every day supplement admission prone to represent no danger of unfavorable health impacts for practically all people in the all inclusive community and isn't intended to apply to individuals under medicinal supervision. Talked about beneath as "sheltered admissions" for grown-ups, most ULs for newborn children, kids, and youths are impressively lower. Average upper admission level (UL) for chose supplements for grown-ups

Vitamin/UL every day

The UL for Vitamin E, niacin, and folic corrosive applies to engineered structures got from supplements or sustained nourishments. The UL for magnesium speaks to allow from a pharmacological specialist in particular and does exclude nourishment or enhancements. As preformed Vitamin An in particular (does exclude beta-carotene).

Source: National Academy of Sciences, Dietary Reference Intakes (1997, 1998, 2000, 2001, and 2002).

calcium	2,500 milligrams
copper	10 milligrams
fluoride	10 milligrams
folic acid	1,000 micrograms
iodine	1,100 micrograms
iron	45 milligrams
magnesium	350 milligrams
manganese	11 milligrams
niacin	35 milligrams
phosphorus	4 grams
selenium	400 micrograms

Vitamin A	micrograms (10,000 IU)
Vitamin C	2,000 milligrams
Vitamin B6	100 milligrams
Vitamin D	50 micrograms (2,000 IU)
Vitamin E	1,000 milligrams
zinc	40 milligrams

Vitamins

Since they can be put away in the liver and fatty tissue, fat-solvent Vitamins, especially Vitamins An and D, have more potential for poisonous quality than do water-dissolvable Vitamins, which, except for Vitamin B12, are promptly discharged in the urine whenever taken in overabundance. Regardless, water-dissolvable Vitamins can be poisonous whenever taken as enhancements or in sustained nourishment. Side effects of intense Vitamin A harming, which normally require a portion of in any event 15,000 µg (50,000 IU) in grown-ups, incorporate stomach torment, sickness, heaving, cerebral pain, dazedness, obscured vision, and absence of solid coordination. Ceaseless hypervitaminosis A, normally coming about because of a continued day by day admission of 30,000 µg (100,000 IU) for a considerable length of time or years, may bring about wide-going impacts, including loss of bone thickness and liver harm. Vitamin A danger in youthful babies might be found in an expanding of the fontanelles (weaknesses) because of expanded intracranial weight. Huge dosages of Vitamin A taken by a pregnant lady likewise can cause formative variations from the norm in a hatchling, particularly whenever taken during the principal trimester; the exact edge for causing birth absconds is obscure, yet under 3,000 μg (10,000 IU) every day gives off an impression of being a protected admission. Albeit most Vitamins happening normally in nourishment don't cause unfriendly impacts, dangerous degrees of Vitamin A might be found in the liver of specific creatures. For instance, early Arctic wayfarers are accounted for to have been harmed by eating polar bear liver. High beta-carotene admission, from supplements or from carrots or different nourishments that are high in beta-carotene, may traceing half a month give a yellowish cast to the skin however doesn't cause indistinguishable poisonous impacts from preformed Vitamin A. High admission of Vitamin D can prompt an assortment of weakening impacts, strikingly calcification of delicate tissues and cardiovascular and renal harm. Despite the fact that not a worry for the vast majority, small kids are particularly helpless against Vitamin D lethality. People with high admissions of braced milk or fish or the individuals who take numerous enhancements may surpass the protected admission of 50 µg (2,000 IU) every day. In light of its capacity as a cancer prevention agent, supplementation with enormous portions (a few hundred milligrams for each day) of Vitamin E in order to protect against coronary illness and other ceaseless maladies has gotten boundless. Such portions—commonly the sum regularly found in nourishment—seem alright for the vast majority, yet their adequacy in counteracting sickness or easing back the maturing procedure has not been illustrated. Day by day admissions more noteworthy than 1,000 mg are not prompted on the grounds that they may meddle with blood thickening, causing hemorrhagic impacts. Huge dosages of niacin (nicotinic corrosive), given for its cholesterol-bringing down impact, may create a blushing of the skin, alongside consuming, shivering, and tingling. Known as a "niacin flush," this is the main marker of niacin overabundance, and this manifestation is the reason for the protected every day admission of 35 mg. Liver poisonous quality and other unfriendly impacts have additionally been accounted for with a few grams of niacin daily. Enormous dosages of Vitamin B6 have been taken in order to treat conditions, for example, carpal passage disorder and premenstrual disorder. The most basic antagonistic impact seen from such supplementation has been a serious tangible neuropathy of the furthest points, including powerlessness to walk. A day by day admission of up to 100 mg is viewed as sheltered, albeit just 1 to 2 mg are required for good health. Utilization of Vitamin C supplements has been broad since 1970, when physicist and Nobel laureate Linus Pauling proposed that the Vitamin was defensive against the normal virus. A few investigations have discovered a moderate advantage of Vitamin C in lessening the length and seriousness of normal cold scenes, however various examinations have neglected to locate a critical impact on occurrence. The most well-known reaction of high Vitamin C admission is looseness of the bowels and other gastrointestinal manifestations, likely due to the unabsorbed Vitamin navigating the digestive system. The sheltered admission of 2,000 mg daily depends on the shirking of these gastrointestinal manifestations. Albeit other conceivable antagonistic impacts of high Vitamin C admission have been researched, none has been shown in sound individuals.

Minerals

An attractive dietary admission of the minerals by and large falls in a genuinely restricted range. In light of connections, a high admission of one mineral may antagonistically influence the assimilation or usage of another. Unreasonable admission from nourishment alone is improbable, yet utilization of strengthened food sources or enhancements expands the opportunity of poisonous quality. Moreover, natural or word related introduction to possibly harmful degrees of minerals displays extra dangers for specific populaces.

Across the board calcium supplementation, essentially by youngsters who don't drink milk and by ladies wanting to avert osteoporosis, has raised worries about conceivable antagonistic results of high calcium consumption. A significant concern has been kidney stones (nephrolithiasis), most of which are made out of a calcium oxalate compound. For quite a long time, a low-calcium diet was suggested for individuals in danger of creating kidney stones, notwithstanding disillusioning viability and a decent lot of research testing the methodology. Notwithstanding, an ongoing report has given solid proof that an eating regimen generally low in sodium and creature protein with typical measures of calcium (1,200 mg for every day) is considerably more viable in avoiding intermittent stone arrangement than was the conventional low-calcium diet. Truth be told, dietary calcium might be defensive against kidney stones since it helps tie oxalate in the digestive system. Clogging is a typical symptom of high calcium admission, however every day utilization of up to 2,500 mg is viewed as safe for grown-ups and for youngsters at any rate one year old. The utilization of magnesium salts in drugs, for example, acid neutralizers and intestinal medicines, may bring about looseness of the bowels, queasiness, and stomach cramps. Debilitated kidney work renders an individual increasingly defenseless to magnesium lethality. Overabundance magnesium admission is impossible from nourishments alone. High-portion iron enhancements, usually used to treat iron lack pallor, may cause blockage and other gastrointestinal impacts. A day by day iron admission of up to 45 mg shows a generally safe of gastrointestinal misery. Intense lethality and passing from ingestion of iron enhancements is a significant harming risk for little youngsters. In individuals with the hereditary issue inherited hemochromatosis, a disease portrayed by the overabsorption of iron, or in the individuals who have rehashed blood transfusions, iron can develop to risky levels, prompting serious organ harm, especially of the liver and heart. It is viewed as judicious for men and postmenopausal ladies to maintain a strategic distance from iron enhancements and high iron admissions from braced nourishments. Poisonous quality from dietary iron has been accounted for in South Africa and Zimbabwe in individuals devouring a conventional brew with an amazingly high iron substance. Overabundance zinc has been accounted for to cause gastrointestinal manifestations, for example, sickness and regurgitating. Interminable admission of a lot of zinc may meddle with the body's usage of copper, hinder invulnerable reaction, and diminish the degree of high-thickness lipoprotein cholesterol (the purported great cholesterol). A sheltered admission of 40 mg of zinc every day is probably not going to be surpassed by nourishment alone, in spite of the fact that it might be surpassed by zinc tablets or enhancements, which are generally utilized regardless of an absence of information about their security or viability. Selenium is poisonous in huge sums. Selenosis (constant selenium lethality) brings about manifestations, for example, gastrointestinal and sensory system unsettling influences, weakness and loss of hair and nails, a garliclike scent to the breath, and skin rash. There additionally have been reports of intense poisonous quality and passing from ingestion of gram amounts of the mineral. Abundance selenium can be destructive whether ingested as selenomethionine, the primary structure found in nourishment, or in the inorganic structures generally found in supplements. An every day admission of up to 400 µg from all sources undoubtedly represents no danger of selenium lethality.

Debilitated thyroid organ capacity, goiter, and other unfriendly impacts may result from high admissions of iodine from nourishment, iodized salt, or pharmaceutical arrangements expected to forestall or treat iodine insufficiency or different issue. Albeit a great many people are probably not going to surpass safe levels, people with specific conditions, for example, immune system thyroid disease, are especially delicate to overabundance iodine admission. While the teeth are creating and before they emit, abundance fluoride ingestion can cause mottled tooth finish; be that as it may, this is just a corrective impact. In grown-ups, abundance fluoride admission is related with impacts running from expanded bone mass to joint agony and solidness and, in extraordinary cases, devastating skeletal fluorosis. Indeed, even in networks where water supplies normally give fluoride levels a few times higher than suggested, skeletal fluorosis is incredibly uncommon. High admissions of phosphorus (as phosphate) may influence calcium digestion unfavorably and meddle with the assimilation of trace components, for example, iron, copper, and zinc. Be that as it may, even with the utilization of phosphate added substances in an assortment of nourishments and in cola refreshments, surpassing safe levels is far-fetched. Manganese harmfulness, with focal sensory system harm and manifestations like Parkinson sickness, is a notable word related risk of breathing in manganese dust, yet once more, it isn't probably going to originate from the eating regimen. So also, copper lethality is probably not going to result from over the top dietary admission, aside from in people with inherited or gained disarranges of copper digestion. The intense impacts of an enormous admission of liquor are notable. Mental impedance begins when the blood focus is about 0.05 percent. A convergence of liquor in the blood of 0.40 percent as a rule causes obviousness, and 0.50 percent can be lethal. Mishaps and viciousness, which are frequently liquor related, are significant reasons for death for youthful people. Ladies who drink during pregnancy chance physical and mental harm to their children (fetal liquor disorder). Liquor additionally can interface perilously with an assortment of prescriptions, for example, sedatives, antidepressants, and torment relievers. Albeit various examinations have affirmed that light to direct consumers have less coronary illness and will in general live longer than either nondrinkers or substantial consumers, expanding interminable liquor utilization conveys with it critical dangers too: liver infection; pancreatitis; suicide; hemorrhagic stroke; mouth, esophageal, liver, and colorectal diseases; and most likely bosom malignancy. In heavy drinkers, dietary debilitation may result from the removal of supplement rich nourishment just as from difficulties of gastrointestinal brokenness and far reaching metabolic adjustments. Thiamin inadequacy, as found in the neurological condition known as Wernicke-Korsakoff disorder, is a sign of liquor addiction and requires dire treatment.

Diet And Chronic Disease

The connection among diet and incessant illness (i.e., a sickness that advances over an all-encompassing period and doesn't resolve unexpectedly) is confused, not just in light of the fact that numerous infections take a very long time to grow yet in addition on the grounds that distinguishing a particular dietary reason is amazingly troublesome. Some planned epidemiologic investigations endeavor to conquer this trouble by traceing subjects for various years. And, after its all said and done, the sheer unpredictability of the eating regimen, just as the multifactorial starting points of interminable illnesses, makes it hard to demonstrate causal connections. Moreover, numerous substances in nourishment seem to act in a synergistic manner—with regards to the entire eating routine instead of as individual specialists—and single-operator studies may miss these intuitive impacts.

CHAPTER ELEVEN

FOOD SUPPLEMENTS

A dietary enhancement is a made item planned to enhance the eating regimen when taken by mouth as a pill, case, tablet, or liquid. An enhancement can give supplements either removed from nourishment sources or manufactured, separately or in blend, so as to expand the amount of their utilization. The class of supplement mixes incorporates nutrients, minerals, fiber, unsaturated fats and amino acids. Dietary enhancements can likewise contain substances that have not been affirmed as being basic to life, however are advertised as having a valuable organic impact, for example, plant colors or polyphenols. Creatures can likewise be a wellspring of supplement fixings, as collagen from chickens or fish. These are additionally sold separately and in blend, and might be joined with supplement fixings. In the United States and Canada, dietary enhancements are viewed as a subset of nourishments, and are controlled likewise. The European Commission has likewise settled orchestrated principles to help protect that nourishment supplements are sheltered and appropriately labeled.

Making an industry assessed to have a 2015

estimation of \$37 billion, there are in excess of 50,000 dietary enhancement items advertised just in the United States, where about half of the American grown-up populace devours dietary enhancements. Multivitamins are the most generally utilized product. For the individuals who neglect to expend a fair diet, the United States National Institutes of Health expresses that specific enhancements "may have value."

In the United States, it is against government guidelines for supplement makers to guarantee that these items forestall or treat any infection. Organizations are permitted to utilize what is alluded to as "Structure/Function" wording if there is substantiation of logical proof for an enhancement giving a potential wellbeing effect. A model would be "______ keeps up sound joints", yet the name must bear a disclaimer that the Food and Drug Administration (FDA) "has not assessed the case and that the dietary enhancement item isn't proposed to "analyze, treat, fix or avoid any disease," in light of the fact that lone a medication can lawfully make such a claim.[8] The FDA authorizes these guidelines, and furthermore forbids the clearance of enhancements and supplement fixings that are perilous, or supplements not made by institutionalized great assembling rehearses (GMPs).

Definition

In the United States, the Dietary Supplement Health and Education Act of 1994 gives this portrayal: "The Dietary Supplement Health and Education Act of 1994 (DSHEA) characterizes the expression "dietary enhancement" to mean an item (other than tobacco) planned to enhance the eating routine that bears or contains at least one of the accompanying dietary fixings: a nutrient, a mineral, a herb or other natural, an amino corrosive, a dietary substance for use by man to enhance the eating routine by expanding the absolute dietary admission, or a concentrate, metabolite, constituent, concentrate, or mix of any of the previously mentioned fixings. Besides, a dietary enhancement must be named as a dietary enhancement and be expected for ingestion and must not be spoken to for use as traditional nourishment or as a sole thing of a supper or of the eating routine. Furthermore, a dietary enhancement can't be endorsed or approved for examination as another medication, anti-toxin, or biologic, except if it was showcased as a nourishment or a dietary enhancement before such endorsement or approval. Under DSHEA, dietary enhancements are regarded to be nourishment, with the exception of motivations behind the medication definition.Per DSHEA, dietary enhancements are expended orally, and are for the most part characterized by what they are not: regular nourishments (counting supper substitutions), restorative foods,[10] additives or pharmaceutical medications. Items proposed for use as a nasal splash, or topically, as a salve applied to the skin, don't qualify. FDA-endorsed drugs can't be fixings in dietary enhancements. Supplement items are or contain nutrients, healthfully basic minerals, amino acids, fundamental unsaturated fats and non-supplement substances separated from plants or creatures or parasites or microscopic organisms, or in the occasion of probiotics, are live microorganisms. Dietary enhancement fixings may likewise be engineered duplicates of normally happening substances (model: melatonin). All items with these fixings are required to be named as dietary supplements. Like nourishments and not at all like medications, no administration endorsement is required to make or sell dietary enhancements; the producer affirms the security of dietary enhancements however the legislature doesn't; and instead of requiring hazard advantage investigation to demonstrate that the item can be sold like a medication, such appraisal is just utilized by the FDA to choose that a dietary enhancement is perilous and ought to be expelled from market.A nutrient is a natural compound required by a life form as a crucial supplement in constrained amounts. A natural concoction compound (or related arrangement of mixes) is known as a nutrient when it can't be combined in adequate amounts by a living being, and should be gotten from the eating routine. The term is restrictive both on the conditions and on the specific living being. For instance, ascorbic corrosive (nutrient C) is a nutrient for humanoid primates, people, guinea pigs and bats, yet not for different warm blooded animals. Nutrient D isn't a basic supplement for individuals who get adequate presentation to bright light, either from the sun or a counterfeit source, as then they incorporate nutrient D in skin. Humans require thirteen nutrients in their eating regimen, the vast majority of which are really gatherings of related atoms, "vitamers", (for example nutrient E incorporates tocopherols and tocotrienols, nutrient K incorporates nutrient K1 and K2). The rundown: nutrients A, C, D, E, K, Thiamine (B1), Riboflavin (B2), Niacin (B3), Pantothenic Acid (B5), Vitamin B6, Biotin (B7), Folate (B9) and Vitamin B12. Nutrient admission underneath prescribed sums can bring about signs and indications related with nutrient insufficiency. There is little proof of advantage when devoured as a dietary enhancement by the individuals who are sound and expending a healthfully sufficient diet.The U.S. Foundation of Medicine sets Tolerable upper admission levels (ULs) for a portion of the nutrients. This doesn't anticipate dietary enhancement organizations from selling items with content per serving higher than the ULs. For instance, the UL for nutrient D is 100 μg (4,000 IU yet items are accessible without solution at 10,000 IU.

Minerals

Minerals are the exogenous concoction components key forever. Four minerals: carbon, hydrogen, oxygen, and nitrogen, are basic forever however are so omnipresent in nourishment and drink that these are not viewed as supplements and there are no suggested admissions for these as minerals. The requirement for nitrogen is tended to by necessities set for protein, which is made out of nitrogen-containing amino acids. Sulfur is basic, however for people, not distinguished as having a prescribed admission as such. Rather, suggested admissions are distinguished for the sulfur-containing amino acids methionine and cysteine. There are dietary enhancements which give sulfur, for example, taurine and methylsulfonylmethane. The basic supplement minerals for people, recorded all together by weight should have been at the Recommended Dietary Allowance or Adequate Intake are potassium, chlorine, sodium, calcium, phosphorus, magnesium, iron, zinc, manganese, copper, iodine, chromium, molybdenum, selenium and cobalt (the last as a part of nutrient B12). There are different minerals which are fundamental for certain plants and creatures, yet might possibly be basic for people, for example, boron and silicon. Fundamental and purportedly basic minerals are advertised as dietary enhancements, separately and in mix with nutrients and different minerals. Despite the fact that when in doubt, dietary enhancement naming and showcasing are not permitted to make disease avoidance or treatment asserts, the U.S. FDA has for certain nourishments and dietary enhancements checked on the science, reasoned that there is huge logical understanding, and distributed explicitly worded permitted wellbeing claims. An underlying decision permitting a wellbeing guarantee for calcium dietary enhancements and osteoporosis was later revised to incorporate calcium supplements with or without nutrient D, viable

January 1, 2010. Instances of permitted wording are demonstrated as traces. So as to meet all requirements for the calcium wellbeing guarantee, a dietary enhancement much contain at any rate 20% of the Reference Dietary Intake, which for calcium implies at any rate 260 mg/serving.

- "Satisfactory calcium all through life, as a feature of a well-adjusted eating regimen, may decrease the danger of osteoporosis."

- "Sufficient calcium as a major aspect of a refreshing eating regimen, alongside physical action, may decrease the danger of osteoporosis in later life."

- "Satisfactory calcium and nutrient D all through life, as a component of a well-adjusted eating routine, may decrease the danger of osteoporosis."

- "Satisfactory calcium and nutrient D as a feature of a refreshing eating regimen, alongside physical action, may decrease the danger of osteoporosis in later life."

Around the same time, the European Food Safety Authority likewise endorsed a dietary enhancement wellbeing guarantee for calcium and nutrient D and the decrease of the danger of osteoporotic breaks by diminishing bone loss. The U.S. FDA likewise affirmed Qualified Health Claims (QHCs) for different wellbeing conditions for calcium, selenium and chromium picolinate. QHCs are upheld by logical proof, however don't meet the more thorough "huge logical understanding" standard required for an approved wellbeing guarantee. In the event that dietary enhancement organizations decide to make such a case, at that point the FDA stipulates the accurate wording of the QHC to be utilized on names and in advertising materials. The wording can be cumbersome: "One examination recommends that selenium admission may diminish the danger of bladder malignant growth in ladies. In any case, one littler examination demonstrated no decrease in chance. In view of these investigations, FDA presumes that it is profoundly dubious that selenium supplements diminish the danger of bladder malignant growth in women."

Proteins and amino acids

Protein-containing supplements, either prepared to-drink or as powders to be blended into water, are promoted as helps to individuals recuperating from sickness or damage, those planning to defeat the sarcopenia of old age, to competitors who accept that strenuous physical action builds protein requirements, to individuals planning to shed pounds while limiting muscle misfortune, i.e., directing a protein-saving altered fast, and to individuals who need to expand muscle size for execution and appearance. Whey protein is a well known ingredient, however items may likewise consolidate casein, soy, pea, hemp or rice protein. As indicated by US and Canadian Dietary Reference Intake rules, the protein Recommended Dietary Allowance (RDA) for grown-ups depends on 0.8 grams protein per kilogram body weight. The suggestion is for inactive and softly dynamic people. Scientific surveys can infer that a high protein diet, when joined with work out, will build bulk and strength, or finish up the opposite. The International Olympic Committee prescribes protein admission focuses for both quality and perseverance competitors at about 1.2-1.8 g/kg weight per day. One audit proposed a most extreme every day protein admission of around 25% of vitality prerequisites, i.e., roughly 2.0 to 2.5 g/kg.A similar protein fixings advertised as dietary enhancements can be joined into dinner substitution and medicinal nourishment items, however those are controlled and marked uniquely in contrast to supplements. In the United

States, "supper substitution" items are nourishments and are named thusly. These commonly contain protein, sugars, fats, nutrients and minerals. There might be content cases, for example, "great wellspring of protein", "low fat" or "lactose free."[33] Medical nourishments, additionally healthfully complete, are intended to be utilized while an individual is under the consideration of a doctor or other authorized human services professional.[34][35] Liquid therapeutic nourishment items - model Ensure - are accessible in normal and high protein renditions. Proteins are chains of amino acids. Nine of these proteinogenic amino acids are viewed as basic for people since they can't be created from different mixes by the human body thus should be taken in as nourishment. Suggested admissions, communicated as milligrams per kilogram of body weight every day, have been established. Other amino acids might be restrictively fundamental for particular ages or ailments. Amino acids, independently and in mixes, are sold as dietary enhancements. The case for enhancing with the stretched chain amino acids leucine, valine and isoleucine is for invigorating muscle protein combination. An audit of the writing finished up this case was unwarranted. In older individuals, supplementation with just leucine brought about an unobtrusive (0.99 kg) increment in slender body mass. The trivial amino corrosive arginine, expended in adequate sums, is thought to go about as a contributor for the blend of nitric oxide, a vasodilator. A survey affirmed circulatory strain lowering. Taurine, a mainstream dietary enhancement fixing with claims made for sports execution, is actually not an amino corrosive. It is combined in the body from the amino corrosive cysteine.

Working out enhancements

This article needs progressively restorative references for check or depends too intensely on essential sources. Working out enhancements are dietary enhancements normally utilized by those associated with lifting weights, weightlifting, blended hand to hand fighting, and sports to encourage an expansion in fit weight. The goal is to build muscle, increment body weight, improve athletic execution, and for certain games, to at the same time decline percent muscle to fat ratio in order to make better muscle definition. Among the most generally utilized are high protein drinks, extended chain amino acids (BCAA), glutamine, arginine, basic unsaturated fats, creatine, HMB, and weight reduction products. Supplements are sold either as single fixing arrangements or as "stacks" – exclusive mixes of different enhancements advertised as offering synergistic focal points. While numerous weight training supplements are additionally devoured by the overall population the recurrence of utilization will contrast when utilized explicitly by muscle heads. One meta-examination reasoned that – for competitors taking an interest in opposition practice preparing and devouring protein supplements for a normal of 13 weeks – complete protein consumption up to 1.6 g/kg of body weight every day would bring about an expansion in quality and without fat mass, yet that higher admissions would not further contribute.

Basic unsaturated fats

Fish oil is a normally utilized unsaturated fat enhancement since it is a wellspring of omega-3 greasy acids. Fatty acids are strings of carbon particles, having a scope of lengths. On the off chance that connections are on the whole single (C-C), at that point the unsaturated fat is called immersed; with one twofold security (C=C), it is called monounsaturated; if there are at least two twofold securities (C=C=C), it is called polyunsaturated. Just two unsaturated fats, both polyunsaturated, are viewed as fundamental to be acquired from the eating regimen, as the others are combined in the body. The "fundamental" unsaturated fats are alpha-linolenic corrosive (ALA), an omega-3 unsaturated fat, and linoleic corrosive (LA), an omega-6 greasy acid. ALA can be prolonged in the body to make other omega-3 unsaturated fats: eicosapentaenoic corrosive (EPA) and docosahexaenoic corrosive (DHA). Plant oils, especially seed and nut oils, contain ALA. Food wellsprings of EPA and DHA are maritime fish, though dietary enhancement sources incorporate fish oil, krill oil and marine green growth removes. The European Food Safety Authority (EFSA) distinguishes 250 mg/day for a consolidated aggregate of EPA and DHA as Adequate Intake, with a suggestion that ladies pregnant or lactating devour an extra 100 to 200 mg/day of DHA. In the United States and Canada are Adequate Intakes for ALA and LA over different phases of life, however there are no admission levels indicated for EPA as well as DHA.

Supplementation with EPA and additionally DHA doesn't seem to influence the danger of death, malignant growth or heart disease. Furthermore, investigations of fish oil supplements have neglected to help cases of averting respiratory failures or strokes. In 2017, the American Heart Association gave a science warning expressing that it couldn't prescribe utilization of omega-3 fish oil supplements for essential aversion of cardiovascular disease or stroke, in spite of the fact that it reaffirmed supplementation for individuals who have a background marked by coronary heart disease.

Normal items

Dietary enhancements can be produced utilizing unblemished sources or concentrates from plants, creatures, green growth, organisms or lichens, including such models as ginkgo biloba, curcumin, cranberry, St. John's wort, ginseng, resveratrol, glucosamine and collagen. Products bearing limited time cases of medical advantages are sold without requiring a remedy in drug stores, general stores, pro shops, military grocery stores, purchasers clubs, direct selling associations, and the internet. While a large portion of these items have a long history of utilization in herbalism and different types of customary medication, concerns exist about their real viability, security and consistency of quality. Canada has distributed a producer and customer control portraying quality, permitting, benchmarks, characters, and normal contaminants of common products. In 2018, offers of home grown enhancements just in the United States were $8.8 billion, with the market developing at about 9% every year, and cannabidiol and mushroom item deals as the highest. Italy, Germany and Eastern European nations were driving shoppers of plant supplements in 2016, with European Union market development gauge to be $8.7 billion by 2020.

Probiotics

In people, the digestive organ is host to in excess of 1,000 types of microorganisms, for the most part microscopic organisms, numbering during the several trillions. "Probiotic" with regards to dietary enhancements is the hypothesis that by orally expending explicit live microbes (or yeast) species, it is conceivable to impact the internal organ microbiota, with subsequent medical advantages. In spite of the fact that there are various asserted advantages of utilizing probiotic supplements, for example, keeping up gastrointestinal wellbeing, to some extent by bringing down danger of and seriousness of obstruction or looseness of the bowels, and improving safe wellbeing, including lower danger of and seriousness of intense upper respiratory tract diseases, i.e., the regular chilly, such claims are not all bolstered by adequate clinical evidence. A survey dependent on interviews with many specialists in microbiome examine communicated worry about "...how biomedical research is co-selected by business elements that spot benefit over health." The worry is convenient, as through 2021, probiotic supplements are relied upon to be the quickest developing portion of the dietary enhancement advertise around the world, while simultaneously, the worldwide medical advantages showcase for probiotic-containing yogurt (a nourishment, not a dietary enhancement) is declining.Likewise with every dietary enhancement, in the United States wrong name wellbeing cases, for example, anticipating or treating illness are restricted by the FDA and tricky promotions by the Federal Trade Commission. Probiotic nourishments and dietary enhancements are permitted to make claims utilizing Structure:Function jargon as long as human preliminary proof is sufficient. In 2005, the FDA gave a Warning Letter to UAS Laboratories for sickness treatment claims (colds, influenza, ulcers, raised blood cholesterol, colon cancer...). The organization reconsidered name and site substance and kept on selling the product. In 2011 the organization was found to have continued the mark and site claims, and the FDA held onto item and halted production. In

2010 a FTC activity was brought against a probiotic nourishment organization for overstated wellbeing claims, bringing about a multimillion-dollar fine and corrections to future advertising. In the European Union a progressively prohibitive methodology has been taken by the EFSA. All proposed wellbeing claims were dismissed in light of the fact that the science was not adequate, and no wellbeing claims are allowed. Nourishments with live microorganisms (yogurt, kefir) can be sold, however without claims.

Probiotic supplements are for the most part viewed as protected. The best concern, prove by audits writing about contextual investigations, is that for individuals with bargained gut divider honesty there might be a danger of foundational disease. Consequently, probiotic look into is required to prohibit microscopic organisms species that are anti-infection resistant.

CHAPTER TWELVE

IMPORTANCE OF NUTRITION

Nourishment is an essential human need and an essential for solid life. A legitimate eating regimen is fundamental from early time of life for development, improvement and dynamic life. Sustenance is the science that manages all the different variables of which nourishment is created and the manner by which appropriate sustenance is achieved.

The normal nourishing prerequisites of gatherings of individuals are fixed and rely upon such quantifiable attributes, for example, age, sex, stature, weight, level of movement and pace of development. In this area traceing are shrouded in detail.

Protein: It's Importance

Proteins are produced using amino acids and they are imperative for living creatures to do a wide scope of capacities fundamental forever. Practically 50% of the protein in our body is as muscles. The nature of protein relies on the substance of basic amino corrosive in the nourishment.

Capacities

Protein as chemicals and hormones is required for a wide scope of imperative metabolic procedures in the body. Proteins supply the weight training material and help body development and advancement in kids and youths. In grown-ups, it keeps up the misfortunes that happen because of mileage. During pregnancy and lactation, extra protein is required for union of fetal and maternal tissue.

Prescribed Dietary Allowance of Proteins

Creature proteins are of higher caliber since they give basic amino acids in right extent. Indeed, even veggie lovers can get enough protein by eating mix of grains, millets, nuts and heartbeats. Milk and egg contain great quality protein. A portion of the rich wellsprings of protein are beats, vegetables, nuts and oil seeds, milk and milk items, meat, fish and poultry. Among the plant nourishments soybean is the most extravagant wellspring of protein, containing over 40% of protein. The measure of protein required for young men (16-18 years) weighing 57 kg weight is 78 gm for every day, while same age bunch young ladies gauging 50 kg need 63 gm/day. Pregnant ladies need 65 gm of protein, while lactating ladies (as long as a half year) need 75 gm/day.

Micronutrients: The Protective Foods

Micronutrients are nutrients and minerals that are required for our body in minute adds up to battle maladies, to help metabolic exercises and secure against contaminations. These are basic for support of wellbeing and life span. Nutrient A: Vitamin A will be a fat-dissolvable nutrient. It has significant job in vision, insusceptible capacities and trustworthiness of skin and bodily fluid film. In India, 3% of school age kids experience the ill effects of nutrient A lack signs like bitot recognizes (a dark fix on the white bit of the eye). Probably the most punctual appearance of nutrient A lack is night visual impairment.

Significance of Vitamin A

Nutrient A is fundamental for typical vision. Its insufficiency brings about night visual impairment and different intricacies. Studies recommend that counteracting nutrient An inadequacy in ladies during and before pregnancy significantly diminishes their danger of mortality and horribleness. Dietary admission of nutrient A is prudent to avert nutrient A lack issue.

Nutrient rich nourishments

Many green verdant vegetables, yellow and orange hued leafy foods are rich wellsprings of beta-carotene.

Professional nutrients like beta carotene are changed over to nutrient A. Just nourishments of creature beginning contain performed nutrient A. Milk and milk items, egg yolk, red palm oil, fish and fish liver oil are likewise plentiful in nutrient A. All out beta-carotene substance of certain groceries.

Nutrient C

Nutrient C is a basic micronutrient and a cancer prevention agent. It gives assurance against diseases. Nutrient C lack causes scurvy portrayed by shortcoming, draining gums and imperfect bone development. Nutrient C helps in wound recuperating, amino corrosive and starch digestion and union of certain hormones. It additionally impacts iron assimilation.

Nutrient C rich nourishments

It is available in all crisp citrus natural products, for example, orange, lemon and amla. Usually devoured organic products, for example, tomato and guava are great wellsprings of nutrient C. Grown grams are likewise rich wellsprings of nutrient C

Iron

Iron is a basic component for the arrangement of

hemoglobin in red platelets and assumes a significant job in transport of oxygen. In our nation, paleness is a significant general medical issue in little youngsters, immature young ladies and pregnant ladies. Around half of the populaces experience the ill effects of healthful weakness. Dietary paleness unfavorably influences work yield among grown-ups and learning capacity in youngsters.

Eat iron-rich nourishments

Plant nourishments like green verdant vegetables, dried foods grown from the ground contain iron and millets, for example, bajra and ragi are great wellsprings of iron. Recall that lone 3-5% of iron from plant sources is consumed by the body. Iron is additionally gotten through meat, fish and poultry items.. Natural products with nutrient C like amla, guava and citrus improve iron retention from plant nourishments. Stay away from tea/espresso after a dinner.

Iodine

Iodine is basic for the combination of thyroid hormones (thyroxin) which thus is liable for ordinary physical and mental development. The day by day necessity of iodine is 100-150 µg/day and it differs with age and certain physiological conditions. Iodine insufficiency issue (IDD) are significant micronutrient lack issue of general wellbeing significance in India. Iodine lack in pregnancy influences the fetal development and its psychological advancement. Iodine lack prompts hypothyroidism, goiter and development impediment. We get iodine from the nourishment we eat particularly ocean nourishments and water Substances considered goitrogens that are available in vegetables like cabbage, cauliflower, custard and so on meddle with metabolic use of iodine. One should utilize iodized salt every day in the eating regimen to avoid IDD.

Immature Growth Spurt

Young people comprise more than one-fifth of India's populace. The word youthful originates from the Latin word 'Puberty' which means to develop, to develop connoting the unique highlights of pre-adulthood.

Development and Nutrition

Sufficient nourishment is basic for development spurt during immaturity. Poor sustenance is frequently refered to as one reason for delay in the beginning of adolescence, particularly among Indian juvenile young ladies. Development spurt that flag the beginning of adolescence relies upon the young lady's achieving a basic load of 30 kg and a basic body piece of 10% muscle to fat ratio. There is an expanded interest for vitality, protein, minerals and nutrients during youthfulness.For what reason do we need vitality? People need sufficient vitality to do their day by day schedule physical work, keep up internal heat level, metabolic movement and to help development. The review led by National Nutrition Monitoring Bureau (NNMB) uncovered that in India about half of people experience the ill effects of constant vitality insufficiency. Vitality necessity of an individual depends on day by day vitality consumption. It is likewise subject to age, body weight, level of physical action, development and physical status. In India, 70-80% of the all out dietary calories are acquired from nourishment grains, for example, oats, millets, heartbeats and tubers. Kids including youths get 55-60% of their day by day prerequisite of calories from starches. Youths require more vitality for sound development. For instance, young ladies and young men in the age gathering of 16-18 require 2060 kcal and 2640 kcal, individually. During pregnancy, extra vitality is expected to help the development of baby and the wellbeing of pregnant ladies. Vitality deficiency prompts under-sustenance and simultaneously overabundance admission brings about weight.

Vitality Rich Food

Incorporate oats, millets, beats, tubers, vegetable oils, ghee, spread, oil seeds, nuts, sugar, jaggery, and so on. Since we get a large portion of our calories from grains, utilization of various assortments of oats and millets ought to be empowered. Coarse oats like jowar and bajra, and millets like ragi are cheap and great wellsprings of vitality

Fat: Human Health

Fat is a significant segment of diet and serves various capacities in our body. It is a concentrated wellspring of vitality giving 9 kcal per gram. Least fat is fundamental to assimilate the fat-solvent nutrients, for example, nutrient A, D, E and K, accessible in the eating routine. Dietary fats are gotten from both plant and creature sources. Vegetable oils are significant dietary wellsprings of basic unsaturated fats (EFA) and other unsaturated fats called MUFAs (monounsaturated unsaturated fats) and PUFAs (polyunsaturated unsaturated fats). Dietary fats give basic unsaturated fats, which are utilitarian parts of layer lipids and have other significant metabolic capacities. Grown-ups need to confine admission of soaked fat (ghee, spread and hydrogenated fat).

Vegetable oils aside from coconut oil are wealthy in unsaturated fats.

Abundance admission of soaked fat things like margarine, ghee, and hydrogenated fat could prompt high blood cholesterol which isn't useful for wellbeing and furthermore it might prompt weight and cardiovascular infection. Fats that are utilized for cooking (vegetable oils, vanaspati, spread and ghee) are named as unmistakable fats. Fats that are available in the nourishment thing are called imperceptible fat. Creature nourishments give high measure of immersed fat.

Suggested Dietary Allowance

Diet for small kids and youthful contains over 25 gm obvious fat. Grown-ups with inactive propensities require 20 gm for every day. Pregnant and lactating ladies need 30 gm for each day of noticeable fat to meet their physiological needs. Linoleic (LIN) linoleinic (LEN) corrosive substance of eatable oils

(g/100 g)

Obesity and Nutrition

Obesity is a state wherein there is a summed up amassing of overabundance fat in fat tissue in the body prompting over 20% of attractive weight. Heftiness has a few antagonistic wellbeing impacts and can even prompt unexpected passing. Stoutness prompts high blood cholesterol, hypertension, coronary illness, diabetes, nerve bladder stone and specific kinds of malignancy.

Causes: Over-eating and decreased physical action together lead to weight. Corpulence and over-weight are brought about by an incessant unevenness between vitality admission and vitality use. High admission of dietary fat likewise causes corpulence. Complex conduct and mental factors likewise cause over-eating and hence lead to corpulence. Metabolic mistakes in vitality usage may support fat amassing. Corpulence in youth and immaturity can prompt grown-up weight. Among ladies, corpulence grows just around pregnancy and after menopause.

How to diminish weight?

- Eat less seared nourishments.

- Eat more leafy foods.

- Eat more fiber-rich nourishment things like entire grains, grams and sprouts.

- Do ordinary exercise to keep the body weight inside typical points of confinement.

- Gradual decrease in body weight is prompted.

- Extreme fasting may prompt wellbeing perils. Appreciate an assortment of nourishments expected to adjust your physical action.

- Eat little dinners consistently at visit interims.

- Chop down sugar, greasy nourishments and liquor.

- Utilize low-fat milk.

- Weight diminishing eating routine must be wealthy in protein and low in sugars and fat.

Nourishment during Pregnancy

Interest for nutritious eating routine is high during pregnancy. Additional nourishment is required to address the issues of the hatchling and the pregnant ladies. In India, it is seen that diets of ladies having a place with the less fortunate gatherings are like non-pregnant and non-lactating ladies in any event, during pregnancy and lactation. Maternal lack of healthy sustenance prompts high commonness of low birth weight babies and high maternal and newborn child mortality. Extra nourishments are required to improve the birth weight and to build mother's muscle to fat ratio stores. Lactating ladies need progressively nutritious nourishment for ideal milk yield.

Dietary necessities of pregnant ladies

Diet of a pregnant lady impacts the heaviness of the infant during childbirth.

Diet during pregnancy ought to contain bigger measures of defensive nourishments.

Pregnant ladies need an extra 300 kcal of vitality, additional 15 gm of protein and 10 gm fat from mid pregnancy onwards.

During pregnancy and lactation extra measure of calcium is required for legitimate arrangement of bone and teeth and furthermore for emission of bosom milk. Iron inadequacy weakness during pregnancy increments maternal mortality and the occurrence of low birth weight. Thus, devouring iron-rich nourishment is fundamental.

Do's and don'ts during pregnancy

- Eat more nourishment during pregnancy and lactation.

- An extra feast is ideal.

- Eat all the more entire grain, grew grams and matured nourishment.

- Take milk/meat/egg.

- Eat a lot of vegetables and organic products.

- Try not to utilize liquor and tobacco.

- Take prescription just when recommended.

- Take iron, folate and calcium supplements normally traceing 14 four months of pregnancy and proceed with the equivalent during lactation.

- Refreshments like tea and espresso tie dietary iron and make it inaccessible; thus they ought to be confined previously and not long after a supper.

- Pregnant ladies need strolling and other physical action and ought to maintain a strategic distance from overwhelming physical work, especially during the most recent month of pregnancy.

What is balance? Basically, it implies eating just as a lot of nourishment as your body needs. You should feel fulfilled toward the finish of a dinner, however not stuffed. For a significant number of us, control implies eating short of what we do now. In any case, it doesn't mean taking out the nourishments you love. Having bacon for breakfast once every week, for instance, could be viewed as control in the event that you tail it with a solid lunch and supper—yet not on the off chance that you tail it with a case of doughnuts and a frankfurter pizza.

Do whatever it takes not to think about specific nourishments as "beyond reach." When you boycott certain food sources, it's normal to need those food sources more, and afterward feel like a disappointment on the off chance that you yield to enticement. Start by lessening segment sizes of unfortunate nourishments and not eating them as frequently. As you diminish your admission of unfortunate nourishments, you may wind up longing for them less or considering them just intermittent extravagances. Think littler segments. Serving sizes have swelled as of late. When eating out, pick a starter rather than a course, split a dish with a companion, and don't structure supersized anything. At home, obvious signals can help with partition sizes. Your serving of meat, fish, or chicken ought to be the size of a deck of cards and a large portion of a cup of pounded potato, rice, or pasta is about the size of a customary light. By serving your dinners on littler plates or in bowls, you can fool your cerebrum into believing it's a bigger bit. On the off chance that you don't feel fulfilled toward the finish of a feast, include increasingly verdant greens or adjust the supper with natural product.

Take as much time as necessary. It's critical to back off and consider nourishment sustenance as opposed to only something to swallow down in the middle of gatherings or while in transit to get the children. It really takes a couple of moments for your cerebrum to tell your body that it has had enough nourishment, so eat gradually and quit eating before you feel full. Eat with others at whatever point conceivable. Eating alone, particularly before the TV or PC, regularly prompts thoughtless indulging. Point of confinement nibble nourishments in the home. Be cautious about the nourishments you keep close by. It's all the more testing to eat with some restraint on the off chance that you have undesirable tidbits and treats primed and ready. Rather, encircle yourself with solid decisions and when you're prepared to remunerate yourself with an extraordinary treat, go out and get it at that point.

Control enthusiastic eating. We don't generally eat just to fulfill hunger. A considerable lot of us additionally go to nourishment to ease pressure or adapt to horrendous feelings, for example, bitterness, dejection, or weariness. Be that as it may, by learning more advantageous approaches to oversee pressure and feelings, you can recapture power over the nourishment you eat and your emotions.

It's what you eat, however when you eat

Have breakfast, and eat littler dinners for the duration of the day. A sound breakfast can kick off your digestion, while eating little, solid dinners keeps your vitality up throughout the day. Abstain from eating late around evening time. Attempt to have supper prior and quick for 14-16 hours until breakfast the traceing morning. Studies recommend that eating just when you're generally dynamic and giving your stomach related framework a long break every day may manage weight

Add more foods grown from the ground to your eating regimen Foods grown from the ground are low in calories and supplement thick, which implies they are pressed with nutrients, minerals, cell reinforcements, and fiber. Concentrate on eating the prescribed day by day measure of at any rate five servings of leafy foods and it will normally top you off and assist you with decreasing unfortunate nourishments. A serving is a large portion of a cup of crude natural product or veg or a little apple or banana, for instance. The majority of us have to twofold the sum we presently eat.

To expand your admission:

Add cancer prevention agent rich berries to your preferred breakfast oat

Eat a variety of sweet natural product—oranges, mangos, pineapple, grapes—for dessert

Swap your typical rice or pasta side dish for a bright serving of mixed greens

Rather than eating handled nibble nourishments, nibble on vegetables, for example, carrots, snow peas, or cherry tomatoes alongside a fiery hummus plunge or nutty spread

Step by step instructions to make vegetables scrumptious

While plain plates of mixed greens and steamed veggies can immediately get flat, there are a lot of approaches to add taste to your vegetable dishes. Include shading. Not exclusively do more brilliant, more profound hued vegetables contain higher centralizations of nutrients, minerals and cancer prevention agents, yet they can change the flavor and make suppers all the more outwardly engaging. Include shading utilizing new or sundried tomatoes, coated carrots or beets, simmered red cabbage wedges, yellow squash, or sweet, vivid peppers. Liven up plate of mixed greens. Branch out past lettuce. Kale, arugula, spinach, mustard greens, broccoli, and Chinese cabbage are altogether pressed with supplements. To add flavor to your plate of mixed greens, take a stab at showering with olive oil, including a zesty dressing, or sprinkling with almond cuts, chickpeas, a little bacon, parmesan, or goat cheddar. Fulfill your sweet tooth. Normally sweet vegetables, for example, carrots, beets, sweet potatoes, yams, onions, ringer peppers, and squash—add sweetness to your suppers and decrease your yearnings for included sugar. Add them to soups, stews, or pasta sauces for a wonderful sweet kick. Cook green beans, broccoli, Brussels sprouts, and asparagus in new ways. Rather than bubbling or steaming these solid sides, have a go at flame broiling, simmering, or sautéing them with bean stew drops, garlic, shallots, mushrooms, or onion. Or then again marinate in tart lemon or lime before cooking.

CHAPTER THIRTEEN

CONCLUSION

Nutrition is the science that interprets the connection of supplements and different substances in nourishment in connection to upkeep, development, multiplication, health and illness of a creature. It incorporates nourishment consumption, retention, absorption, biosynthesis, catabolism and excretion.The eating routine of a life form is the thing that it eats, which is to a great extent dictated by the accessibility and attractiveness of nourishments. For people, a solid eating regimen incorporates arrangement of nourishment and capacity techniques that safeguard supplements from oxidation, warmth or filtering, and that lessens danger of foodborne ailments. A kind of sugar, dietary fiber, for example non-edible material, for example, cellulose, is required, for both mechanical and biochemical reasons, in spite of the fact that the precise reasons stay vague. A few supplements can be put away - the fat-solvent vitamins - while others are required pretty much constantly. Unexpected weakness can be brought about by an absence of required supplements, or for certain vitamins and minerals, an over the top required supplement.The human body requires seven significant sorts of supplements. Not all supplements give vitality but rather are as yet significant, for example, water and fiber. Micronutrients are significant however required in littler sums. Vitamins are basic natural aggravates that the human body can't combine. As atomic science, organic chemistry, and hereditary qualities advance, nourishment has gotten increasingly centered around digestion and metabolic pathways - biochemical strides through which substances inside us are changed starting with one structure then onto the next. The macronutrients are starches, fiber, fats, protein, and water. The macronutrients (barring fiber and water) give auxiliary material (amino acids from which proteins are manufactured, and lipids from which cell films and some flagging particles are assembled) and vitality.Nutritional Disorders are caused by the lack of certain food nutrients in the body which are injurious to health and may be deadly in many cases. Nutritional Disorders covers for malnutrition, and excess intake of the nutrition which may also hamper health in different ways.It's not only what we eat, it also covers for how we eat it and what quantity of food we take these nutrients. It's beneficial when we eat some amount of food in certain quantities (g or mg) to allow adequate metabolism and good digestion of the foods.